Perfect Pregnancy

June Thompson

Consulting Editors
Allen H. Babbitz, M.D.
Gila Leiter, M.D.

BEECHWOOD
HEALTHBOOKS

Beechwood Healthbooks Inc
2026 Beechwood, Wilmette, IL 60091

Published in the United States by
Beechwood Healthbooks Inc
2026 Beechwood,
Wilmette, IL 60091

ISBN 0-916363-15-5 Second Printing, AAL

Project Editor Esther Labi

Designer Philip Letsu

Managing Editor Lindsay McTeague

Editorial Director Sophie Collins

Art Director Sean Keogh

Production Nikki Ingram

Developmental Editors David Manhoff,
Cary Barbor

Note: The terms "he" and "she," used in alternate
sections, refer to people of both sexes, unless a
topic or sequence of photographs applies only to a
man or woman.

Printed in China

Reviewers

Gila Leiter, M.D.
Dr. Leiter is Assistant Clinical Professor, Mount
Sinai School of Medicine, New York, and has a
private practice in Park Avenue, New York. She is
a fellow of the American College of Obstetrics and
Gynecology and a certified member of the
American Board of Obstetrics and Gynecology.
She has four children.

Allen H. Babbitz, M.D., FACOG
Dr. Babbitz is a graduate of the University of
Wisconsin at the Medical School. He has practiced
Obstetrics and Gynecology for 23 years in
Milwaukee, Wisconsin. He is a clinical associate
professor of OB/GYN at the UW Medical School,
and a clinical assistant professor at the Medical
College of Wisconsin.

Preface

This book is intended to provide general
information concerning pregnancy. It is not
intended to replace consultation with your doctor
or health care professional. Many hours have been
spent checking and rechecking the medicines,
treatment, and procedures to assure accuracy.
Unfortunately, some changes in obstetrics do
occur. Please consult your doctor or health care
professional if you have any questions.

Notice

The author and publisher of this book have taken
care to make certain that all medical techniques
and references are correct, and compatible with
national standards generally accepted at
the time of publication. The author
and publisher disclaim any liability,
loss, injury, or damage incurred as a
consequence, directly or indirectly,
of the use and application of the
contents of this book.

INDEX

(See also technical terms on p. 83)

USING THIS BOOK

This guide is divided into six subject areas: 1 Conception; 2 Health and Diet; 3 Exercise and Relaxation; 4 Prenatal Care, Labor, and Birth; 5 You and Your Baby; 6 Your Personal File. If you know which subject area you wish to access, turn to the relevant tab. On each tab you will find a detailed table of the contents of that section of the guide. If you are unsure where to find the information you need, turn to the alphabetical index on page 3.

Subject heading
Each double-page spread is self-contained, to give a concise treatment of a subject's major points of interest.

Introduction
Running text gives a brief overview of the subject under discussion, highlighting important factors, common problems, and easy solutions.

Tab
Color-coded subject dividers enable you to turn quickly and easily to the section you need. Each divider offers a contents listing of the subjects included on pages that bear the same colored band.

Boxed information
Subjects of related interest and quick-reference charts appear in colored boxes, enhancing reference value and making the text more user-friendly.

Numbered points
Easy-to-follow sequences of step-by-step words and photographs explain all aspects of pregnancy.

Color photographs
A combination of practical and inspirational photographs and illustrations complement the informative text.

Conception

CONCEPTION

Deciding to have a baby is one of the most important decisions that you and your spouse will ever make. Healthy parents are more likely to have healthy babies, so the healthier you are before you conceive and the healthier you remain during pregnancy, the better it will be for your own wellbeing and that of your baby.

Pregnancy and childbirth have never been safer in the developed world, but ensuring you are in good shape will make it easier for you to cope with pregnancy, the delivery, and the demands of a new baby. Preparing for pregnancy should begin at least three months before you start trying to conceive. To help you prepare, this section looks at the steps you should take to plan your pregnancy and the questions you may ask.

PLANNING AHEAD

By planning your preconceptual program, you and your spouse can make sure you are in the best of health and are aware of any potential hazards or hereditary factors that could affect your health and that of your baby. There are a number of steps you and your partner should take at least three months before trying to conceive.

REVIEW YOUR LIFESTYLE AND GENERAL HEALTH

■ Do you smoke cigarettes, drink alcohol, or use drugs such as marijuana, cocaine, or heroin? If so, you can seriously harm yourself and your baby. See pp. 10–11 for advice on changing your habits.

■ Are you reasonably fit? If not, see pp. 44–47 for improving your fitness.

■ What is your general health and immunization status? For advice on health and immunization checks see pp. 8–9. Discuss any problems with your doctor.

REVIEW YOUR NUTRITION

■ Are you overweight or underweight? Being significantly over- or underweight may reduce your chances of conceiving (see p. 11).

■ Do you eat fewer than three meals a day, or constantly snack? Do you eat a special diet? Eating a balanced diet is essential for a healthy baby. See pp. 28–29 for advice about nutrition.

STOP USING CONTRACEPTION

■ If you use an intrauterine device (IUD), have it removed before you plan to become pregnant, since it can increase the risk of a intrauterine infection.

■ Stop using the contraceptive pill at least three menstrual cycles before trying to conceive. It may take a few months for "natural" periods to resume, and there is also evidence that the pill can affect the absorption of certain vitamins and minerals.

■ Use natural family-planning methods or a barrier method in the fertile period instead.

ARE YOU AT RISK FROM ANIMALS OR FOOD?

■ Do you have a cat or live on a farm? Do you eat raw meat, eat unpasteurized or mold-ripened cheeses, or drink unpasteurized milk? You could contract an infection from these foods or animals that could harm your baby. See pp. 24–25 for advice on how to help avoid the danger.

HAZARDS IN YOUR HOME AND AT WORK

Before you conceive, check your exposure to pollutants, which can affect your unborn baby or may lead to a miscarriage.

Health hazards at work

Try to find out about hazards at work, such as chemicals, gases, or radiation from radioactive materials or X-ray equipment. Recent studies about the harmful effects on the fetus of visual display terminals (VDT) have found no evidence of any risk, but you may wish to reduce your daily exposure. Talk to your employer if you have any concerns about your safety at work. (See also p. 25 for further advice on safeguarding your health at work when pregnant.)

Chemicals to avoid

Mercury may be found in tuna fish, agricultural chemicals, weedkillers, and dental amalgam fillings. Avoid eating too much tuna, handling weedkillers or insecticides for pest control, and using cleaning products that may be toxic.

Lead can be found in:

■ Drinking water: If you live in a house with old pipes, you may have unacceptable levels of lead in your water. Ask your local utility company to test your drinking water. In the meantime, filter your water.

■ Old flaking paint: You may wish to have this tested by a professional lead inspector. If you decide to remove old paint, have it done professionally and stay away from the area while the work is going on.

■ Fuel: Avoid exposure to gasoline that is not unleaded.

RESPONSIBLE FATHERHOOD

Giving your baby a good start in life is dependent on your own health as well as your spouse's. You produce sperm all the time, although they take 100 days to mature fully. During that time the quantity and quality of the sperm can be affected by:

■ Excessive alcohol and smoking

■ Drugs

■ Poor nutrition

■ Obesity

■ Stress

■ Environmental pollution, including exposure to chemicals and toxins.

PRECONCEPTION CHECKS

Before you conceive, your doctor will check your health in a variety of ways. These include taking your full medical and obstetric history, establishing whether you have had childhood diseases such as chicken pox, or any sexually transmitted diseases, and checking your immunity to rubella (German measles). You should be offered advice about any medical problems you may have, such as high blood pressure or diabetes, since some conditions require special attention during pregnancy. Your doctor will talk to you about genetic testing, should you require it, and it is also essential that you check with him about any prescribed or nonprescription medications you take, to make sure they will be safe for you and your baby while you are pregnant.

CHECK ANY MEDICAL CONDITIONS

Do you have or have you ever had:
- A medical condition such as asthma, diabetes, high blood pressure, epilepsy, or a family history of these?
- A history of miscarriages?
- A sexually transmitted disease such as herpes, chlamydia, or gonorrhea?

Many women with medical conditions have a routine pregnancy. Sometimes, however, problems can arise, and special precautions may be necessary. To reduce the risk of complications, you should review your full medical history with your doctor before you become pregnant. Precautions or treatment can then be recommended if necessary. Do not stop taking any medicines unless advised by your doctor.

CHECK YOUR IMMUNIZATION STATUS

- Have you been immunized against infectious diseases such as rubella (German measles) or measles?
- Do you plan to travel to a foreign country when pregnant?

Although childhood infectious diseases are rare during pregnancy, if you catch rubella in early pregnancy, or chicken pox around the time of birth, your baby may suffer serious complications. Your immunity can be tested by a simple blood test. If necessary, you can be immunized against rubella, but you will be advised to wait three months after the vaccination before conceiving. Many doctors also advise updating immunizations for other diseases such as mumps, hepatitis B, and tetanus. If you plan to travel or live in a foreign country while pregnant, certain other immunizations such as yellow fever or typhoid and antimalaria medications may be recommended. Because some shots cannot be given to pregnant women, or take time to administer, check with your doctor and plan ahead if you are going to need them. Women who will be in or beyond their 14th week of pregnancy during flu season should be vaccinated against influenza. Check with your doctor.

REVIEW YOUR FAMILY HISTORY

Although it is not possible to cure many birth defects, or even to prevent them (some of the most common are still chance events), breakthroughs have been made in identifying those people at risk of having a child with an abnormality and of screening them for those abnormalities. In some cases, two parents need to have the gene for the baby to have the disorder; in others, only one affected parent can pass the trait onto the baby. If there is anyone who suffers from one of these conditions in the close family of you or your spouse (parent, brother and sister, first cousin), it is worth seeking help before you try to conceive:

■ Genetic disorders such as cystic fibrosis, sickle cell anemia, thalassemia or Tay-Sachs disease.

■ Birth defects such as Down's syndrome, Turner syndrome, congenital heart defects, cleft palate, or hare lip.

Genetic screening or counseling involves taking you and your spouse's complete medical and family history and calculating the risk of your passing a trait onto your baby. If the odds of your baby being affected by a serious defect are higher than you consider acceptable, you may be able to consider in vitro fertilization (IVF) using donated eggs or sperm, or adoption.

SCREENING TESTS FOR GENETIC DISORDERS

■ Screening of genetic disorders such as those mentioned above can be carried out with special blood tests on both partners. If both are found to be carriers, each child will have a one in four chance of being affected with the disease.

■ Some disorders are linked mainly to specific ethnic groups. For instance, sickle cell disease occurs more frequently among people of African or Caribbean origin; thalassemia among those of Mediterranean and Southeast Asian descent, and Tay-Sachs disease among Ashkenazi Jews.

■ If you are a carrier of the sickle cell or thalassemia trait, you will not have the condition and its presence will not affect you during your pregnancy.

Other tests

Other tests you might like to consider include a test for blood type and antibody screening, especially if you have had a transfusion or are Rh negative (see pp. 64–65). You could also test for immunity to toxoplasmosis, which may occur if your diet includes undercooked meat (see pp. 24–25).

DENTAL CHECKS

Although you should continue to visit your dentist during pregnancy, have a dental check before you conceive. This will help ensure that your teeth and gums are healthy during pregnancy and avoid the need for any X rays while you are pregnant. You may also wish to have any fillings containing mercury changed. Don't forget to remind the dentist of your condition if you visit while you are pregnant.

CHANGING YOUR HABITS

Being under- or overweight, smoking, and excessive alcohol and drug intake can reduce your chances of conceiving. Both spouses should take steps to change their habits before you try to become pregnant.

WHY STOP SMOKING OR TAKING DRUGS?

There is lots of evidence to show that smoking is harmful to your baby before, during, and after birth, since it lowers the amount of oxygen and nourishment the baby receives. The risks of smoking on your baby's health include:

- Lower birthweight, which increases the likelihood of suffering illness
- Increased likelihood of miscarriage or stillbirth
- Increased likelihood of death by sudden infant death syndrome
- Increased likelihood of respiratory infections, asthma, and ear infections
- Likelihood of being shorter than children of nonsmoking parents.

Nicotine patches and nicotine gum can be helpful in stopping smoking, but are not recommended for use in pregnancy.

Taking drugs such as cocaine or heroin during pregnancy puts your baby at risk for problems such as miscarriage, prematurity, or stillbirth. It may also be born addicted to the drug. To be weaned off drugs, ask your doctor to refer you for specialized help or look in the phone book for an organization that can help.

ALCOHOL

Alcohol in your bloodstream can cross the placenta and enter your baby's bloodstream. Heavy drinking can lead to a miscarriage in the early stages of pregnancy or have a damaging effect on your baby's health, including mental retardation. Babies of heavy drinkers may be born with a range of physical and mental problems known as fetal alcohol syndrome. Babies with this syndrome are shorter and lighter in weight than normal babies, have small heads, abnormal features, and are usually mentally handicapped. They may also be hyperactive and have severe behavioral problems.

- The amount you drink can reduce your fertility and ability to conceive.
- The safest approach is to stop drinking altogether while you try to conceive and when you are pregnant. Otherwise, reduce your alcohol consumption to not more than one or two drinks (see below) once or twice a week.
- Getting drunk or binge drinking is particularly dangerous.

One drink of alcohol equals half a pint of beer, a glass of wine, or one shot of alcohol.

INCREASE YOUR FOLIC ACID INTAKE

■ Scientific studies have found that increasing your levels of folic acid in the 12 weeks before and after conception can significantly reduce the risk of your baby being born with defects of the brain and spinal cord, such as spina bifida.

■ Folic acid is one of the B vitamins. Good sources include green leafy vegetables; whole-wheat bread and fortified cereals; oranges and bananas; milk, yogurt, and cheese; beans and legumes such as black-eyed peas and lentils.

■ It is generally recommended that you take a supplement of between 0.4mg (400 micrograms) to 1mg of folic acid daily in tablet form before you try to conceive and for the first 12 weeks of pregnancy. If you already have a child born with defects of the brain and spinal cord, you may be required to increase this dose.

CHECK YOUR WEIGHT

Being significantly under- or overweight may reduce your chances of conceiving. The health of your baby is also influenced by your weight.

■ If you are underweight because you are not eating enough, you could be low in vital nutrients such as vitamins, iron, and calcium, which can affect both your own and your baby's health.

■ If you are so underweight that your periods have stopped or are irregular, you are unlikely to conceive until your weight is more normal.

■ If you are seriously underweight or suffer from an eating disorder such as bulimia or anorexia, seek professional advice because these conditions can cause growth problems in the developing fetus.

■ If you are overweight, you are at risk of raised blood pressure, which may be a problem in late pregnancy. You may also be at risk for "gestational" diabetes, that is, diabetes developed during pregnancy. The extra weight can also put an increased strain on your joints during pregnancy and lead to a worsening of common problems such as backache and breathlessness.

■ Dieting during pregnancy is not normally recommended, so if you need to lose weight, do it before you try to conceive. You should aim to lose weight slowly and steadily, following a healthy eating plan and by taking moderate exercise. Avoid crash diets because they can deprive your body of essential nutrients and harm your health. Ask your doctor or a dietitian for further advice.

RESPONSIBLE FATHERHOOD

Smoking or moderate to heavy drinking may cause fertility problems, and your spouse's health may be harmed by her breathing in your cigarette smoke. Fathers who drink heavily also have a higher risk of producing a child with fetal alcohol syndrome. Like your wife, you should give up smoking and stop drinking or reduce your alcohol intake before you try to conceive. Some medications, as well as drugs such as marijuana, may lower your sperm count.

CONCEPTION

If you and your spouse have been following the preconception guidelines in this section (see pp. 6–11) for at least three months before trying to conceive, you have given yourself an excellent chance of conceiving and producing a healthy baby.

FOR A PREGNANCY TO OCCUR

- The woman must be ovulating (see right).
- Intercourse must take place close to ovulation.
- There must be an adequate number of good-quality active sperm reaching the egg, including one to fertilize it.
- There must not be any barrier to prevent fertilization from taking place.
- Once fertilization has occurred, the developing embryo needs to become successfully embedded in the prepared lining of the uterus.

OVERCOMING PROBLEMS WITH CONCEPTION

Don't be disappointed if conception does not occur immediately after you have unprotected intercourse. Studies have found that only one in five couples with no barrier to fertility conceive within a month. If after trying to become pregnant for a year you are still unsuccessful, talk to your doctor who can arrange tests. These can include tests to confirm ovulation, infection screening, or checking the Fallopian tubes for blockages.

RESPONSIBLE FATHERHOOD

Tight slacks or underwear can raise the temperature of the testicles and inhibit sperm production, so change to boxer shorts. Follow the general guidelines to help conception such as eating healthily, reducing obesity, and stopping smoking.

WHEN DO YOU OVULATE?

A woman is born with about 250,000 to 400,000 immature eggs (ova) in each ovary. About 14 days before a period is due, an egg ripens and is released into the Fallopian tube. This is known as ovulation. Once the egg is released, it lives for up to 24 hours, although a sperm can live inside a woman's body for up to 72 hours, or even 6–7 days in some cases. The menstrual cycle generally averages 28 days, but many women have irregular cycles, irregular ovulation, or other problems. So establishing that ovulation takes place and pinpointing when, can be crucial to successful conception. This can be done by:

■ Body temperature monitoring – the "temperature method"

Record your temperature on a chart every day over the course of a month. After ovulation has occurred, the body temperature rises by up to 1°F (0.5°C). As the temperature rises only after ovulation has taken place, it cannot be used to detect ovulation, and intercourse must take place as soon as possible after the rise has been noted. Difficulties in reading and interpretation can impair the reliability of this method.

■ Cervical mucus changes

At the beginning and end of the cycle, the mucus is scant, sticky, and opaque. As the estrogen level peaks, just before ovulation, it gets profuse, slick, and glassy. This fertile mucus is favorable to the sperm and so to fertilization. This information is often used in conjunction with the temperature method.

■ Home ovulation prediction tests

Prior to ovulation, the amount of a substance known as luteinizing hormone (LH) in a woman's body increases sharply. Home ovulation prediction tests work by detecting the amount of LH in a woman's urine on a number of days during her menstrual cycle – a definite increase shows that the time of peak fertility is approaching. Having sexual intercourse in the one to two days following the detection of the LH surge will improve your chances of becoming pregnant. These home prediction tests are available from pharmacies.

SIGNS OF PREGNANCY

There are a number of signs and symptoms that can indicate that you are pregnant. You may not notice all of them at first, or you may know you are pregnant because you "feel different." A missed period is the most obvious sign that you are pregnant, especially if your periods are usually regular. But there may be other early indications, including a frequent need to urinate and tender or enlarged breasts.

Sensitivity to smells
You may have a increased sensitivity to strong smells, such as cigarette smoke or certain foods, and they may make you feel sick.

Breast changes
High levels of progesterone and estrogen (see p. 23) may make your breasts feel heavy and tender. Your nipples may also become slightly darker.

Missed periods
A period is a sign that the womb does not need the extra lining it has prepared in case it needs to receive a fertilized egg. So a missed period may mean that fertilization has taken place.

Frequent need to urinate
This is due to the hormone relaxin (see p. 23) relaxing the bladder muscles, combined with increased fluids in the body and increased urine production.

Fatigue
You may feel very tired due to the rapidly growing placenta and fetus, and hormonal changes.

Taste changes
Hormonal changes may make some foods taste bad, or leave a metallic taste in the mouth. You may also start to crave certain foods.

Morning sickness
Rapidly rising levels of of the hormone HCG (see p. 23), increased stomach acid, and an increased sensitivity to smells may contribute to nausea and vomiting.

Increased vaginal discharge
This is due to hormonal changes.

CONFIRMING THE PREGNANCY

■ Early confirmation of pregnancy is important so that you can make any necessary changes to your lifestyle as soon as possible. If your pregnancy is planned, you should already be eating healthily, exercising regularly, and working to cut out any bad habits such as smoking or drinking. If your pregnancy is not planned, it is important to make these changes now.

■ If your period is late and you have any of the other signs of pregnancy described opposite, a urine or blood test can be carried out to confirm the diagnosis.

■ You can do a urine test yourself at home, using a kit that you can buy from your drugstore. Alternatively, your doctor can test your urine for you.

■ Your doctor may also offer you a blood test to confirm your pregnancy. This is more sophisticated than a urine test and measures precisely the amount of the hormone human chorionic gonadotrophin (HCG, see p. 23) circulating in the blood. Because the amount of HCG varies throughout pregnancy, it also helps to pinpoint the date when conception occurred and to predict when your baby is due (see p. 20 for more details of this). In some states in the U.S., you may also be asked if you wish to take an HIV test, but you cannot be forced to have one.

■ Once you are more than six weeks pregnant, your doctor may follow a urine or blood test with a medical examination. He or she may examine the uterus, which will feel enlarged and softened, by gently pressing your abdomen or by an internal examination.

HOME-TESTING KITS

Your pregnancy can be diagnosed from the first day of your missed period (about two weeks after conception if you have a regular menstrual cycle) using a pregnancy testing kit. These are simple and quick to use and can be bought from your local drugstore.

■ It is best to test your urine first thing in the morning before you have drunk anything, since this is usually the time that the urine contains the highest amount of HCG.

■ If the instructions are followed correctly, the test should give an accurate result.

■ Occasionally, a test may give a "false negative"; that is, it may tell you that you are not pregnant even though you are. This is more likely if your periods are irregular.

■ If your result is negative but your period has still not arrived one week later, try the test again.

■ If your urine test is positive, you should consult your doctor as soon as possible.

CHOOSING A PRACTITIONER

Now that you are pregnant, you and your spouse will need to decide how to prepare for childbirth, where you want the baby delivered, and by whom. There are several options available. For instance, do you want your leading doctor to be an obstetrician? Is the doctor's practice near your home or work? What is his or her attitude to your concerns about active childbirth, pain relief in labor, the presence of fathers at the delivery, and breastfeeding? When making your decision, think about your basic approach to pregnancy and the style and type of care and delivery that you want.

YOUR FAMILY PHYSICIAN

Your family physician may be able to provide most of your prenatal care, with hospital appointments being necessary only for special tests or if complications arise. The advantage is that your physician knows you personally and knows your medical history. Not all family physicians offer obstetric care, however, and your doctor may refer you to an obstetrician they know and respect.

CHOOSING AN OBSTETRICIAN

Obstetricians are doctors who specialize in the care of pregnant women, and are trained to handle any complications of pregnancy and delivery. If yours is a high-risk pregnancy (for example, if you have a history of miscarriages, or a medical condition such as diabetes), you will need to see an obstetrician. Even if you have no such complications, you can, if you wish, see an obstetrician from the start. Before choosing an obstetrician, it is best to ask friends and acquaintances for a personal recommendation and then discuss this with your doctor. Alternatively, you can ask your doctor to refer you to someone.

MIDWIFERY CARE

Midwives are highly trained to provide a woman with continuing health care from early pregnancy right through labor, delivery, and the early days after birth. Before being allowed to practice, a midwife must, by law, be registered. Most are also trained nurses. A midwife may work in the community with a family doctor, or in a hospital. There are also some independent midwives. A community or independent midwife is likely to get to know you well and help you to plan the kind of care that you would like. Some hospitals are also introducing "one to one" midwifery care. If any complications arise at any time, the midwife will refer you to your family doctor or obstetrician.

CHOOSING THE PLACE OF BIRTH

Choosing the place of birth will inevitably depend to some extent on the choices available in your area or the hospital from where your obstetrician practices. This may be a large general hospital with a specialized maternity unit or a birthing room. A birthing room provides a comfortable setting similar to a bedroom or hotel room, but it is fully equipped to allow a mother to stay in the same bed from labor through delivery to postpartum care. Other alternatives include a birth unit within a small community hospital, a birth center that is not in or near a general hospital, or a home birth. Home births are not normally recommended for first babies.

PRENATAL CLASSES

Attending a prenatal class can be of great benefit to you and your spouse. At most classes you will learn about the changes to your mind and body you can expect during pregnancy. You will learn what happens during labor so you can be more prepared and consequently more relaxed and able to deal with pain. Some aspects of early parenthood will also usually be covered. Classes offer an opportunity to make new friends and obtain emotional support from other pregnant women. Before deciding which approach is right for you and what class to attend, it is best to read as much as you can and obtain more specific information from the instructor of any class you are thinking of attending.

THE PURPOSE OF PRENATAL CLASSES

Whether they are called prenatal or childbirth classes, these types of classes usually include information about preparation for childbirth, relaxation techniques for coping with labor, the physical process of labor, information about various birth methods and pain relief, and preparation for parenthood. Videos on labor and various birth methods may also be shown.

Some classes will discuss early pregnancy concerns such as nutrition, exercises, and fetal development – although many women do not start attending prenatal classes until the sixth or seventh month of pregnancy – and all should give you the opportunity to ask questions and talk about any worries you may have. If your class is in or near the hospital where you plan to give birth, you will be able to get more specific information about the practices and facilities there, and arrange a tour of the hospital.

Most classes also encourage spouses to attend. If you aren't married or your husband is unable or unwilling to attend, you may be able to take a friend or relative along with you if you wish. If you have chosen someone other than your husband to be your birth companion, they will be made welcome at classes.

FINDING THE RIGHT CLASS FOR YOU

Allow yourself enough time to find the right class. Classes may be run by a nurse at a health center, doctor's clinic, or the hospital you are attending for your prenatal care. Or you may prefer a class run by a government or volunteer organization, or by a private childbirth teacher or counselor. Classes close to where you work may fit your schedule better; those closer to home mean that you will meet parents and babies who are likely to live close by, which will make keeping in touch after the birth easier.

Once you've chosen the type of class you want to attend or have heard of one that is good, you may want to reserve a place in advance – if it is very popular, there may not be an immediate vacancy. Classes typically meet once a week for about two hours and last for around eight to ten weeks. Aim to have completed a course with about four weeks to spare before your due date.

TYPES OF CLASSES

You can, if you wish, go to more than one type of class – for example, an exercise class for pregnant women, as well as a more conventional prenatal one. Or you may prefer one that practices special birth techniques or follows a particular philosophy or school of thought. No childbirth class should promise you a painfree labor or delivery, but there are several relaxation methods or philosophical approaches available which may help you to avoid or minimize the use of drugs. However, you do not have to follow one approach only. Many classes combine the best elements of various philosophies.

COMMON PRENATAL APPROACHES

Robert Bradley

This American obstetrician invented the "husband-coached" approach to childbirth, in which the man acts as the woman's coach and supporter in pregnancy. A healthy diet and exercise are emphasized to ease discomforts of pregnancy, and deep breathing is advocated for a drugfree labor.

Fernand Lamaze

Lamaze was a French doctor who developed an approach centered on techniques of breathing relaxation. He believed that the pain of childbirth was heightened by fear and tension and that pregnant women could be conditioned by practicing relaxation techniques to respond to pain in a positive way. This approach has now become more flexible, and women should not feel that something is going wrong if they have pain in labor.

Active birth

This approach, based on yoga, involves moving around and changing positions throughout labor. You give birth in a squatting or kneeling position, or on all fours, while your husband or birth partner supports you physically. It is important to learn stretching exercises and how to adopt "open" positions.

WHEN IS YOUR BABY DUE?

To calculate when your baby is due, use the calendar below. Look along the top rows to find the first day of your last period; the date below it is your estimated date of delivery (EDD). In the example below, if the first day of your last period was January 14, then your estimated due date would be October 21. Remember, though, that only five percent of babies are born on their due date. It is perfectly normal for babies to be born two weeks before or two weeks after the EDD.

Date of your last period
Estimated date of delivery

Jan	1 2 3 4 5 6 7 8 9 10 11 12 13 14 15 16 17 18 19 20 21 22 23 24 25 26 27 28 29 30 31
Oct	8 9 10 11 12 13 14 15 16 17 18 19 20 21 22 23 24 25 26 27 28 29 30 31 1 2 3 4 5 6 7

Feb	1 2 3 4 5 6 7 8 9 10 11 12 13 14 15 16 17 18 19 20 21 22 23 24 25 26 27 28
Nov	8 9 10 11 12 13 14 15 16 17 18 19 20 21 22 23 24 25 26 27 28 29 30 1 2 3 4 5

March	1 2 3 4 5 6 7 8 9 10 11 12 13 14 15 16 17 18 19 20 21 22 23 24 25 26 27 28 29 30 31
Dec	6 7 8 9 10 11 12 13 14 15 16 17 18 19 20 21 22 23 24 25 26 27 28 29 30 31 1 2 3 4 5

April	1 2 3 4 5 6 7 8 9 10 11 12 13 14 15 16 17 18 19 20 21 22 23 24 25 26 27 28 29 30
Jan	6 7 8 9 10 11 12 13 14 15 16 17 18 19 20 21 22 23 24 25 26 27 28 29 30 31 1 2 3 4

May	1 2 3 4 5 6 7 8 9 10 11 12 13 14 15 16 17 18 19 20 21 22 23 24 25 26 27 28 29 30 31
Feb	5 6 7 8 9 10 11 12 13 14 15 16 17 18 19 20 21 22 23 24 25 26 27 28 1 2 3 4 5 6 7

June	1 2 3 4 5 6 7 8 9 10 11 12 13 14 15 16 17 18 19 20 21 22 23 24 25 26 27 28 29 30
March	8 9 10 11 12 13 14 15 16 17 18 19 20 21 22 23 24 25 26 27 28 29 30 31 1 2 3 4 5 6

July	1 2 3 4 5 6 7 8 9 10 11 12 13 14 15 16 17 18 19 20 21 22 23 24 25 26 27 28 29 30 31
April	7 8 9 10 11 12 13 14 15 16 17 18 19 20 21 22 23 24 25 26 27 28 29 30 1 2 3 4 5 6 7

Aug	1 2 3 4 5 6 7 8 9 10 11 12 13 14 15 16 17 18 19 20 21 22 23 24 25 26 27 28 29 30 31
May	8 9 10 11 12 13 14 15 16 17 18 19 20 21 22 23 24 25 26 27 28 29 30 31 1 2 3 4 5 6 7

Sept	1 2 3 4 5 6 7 8 9 10 11 12 13 14 15 16 17 18 19 20 21 22 23 24 25 26 27 28 29 30
June	8 9 10 11 12 13 14 15 16 17 18 19 20 21 22 23 24 25 26 27 28 29 30 1 2 3 4 5 6 7

Oct	1 2 3 4 5 6 7 8 9 10 11 12 13 14 15 16 17 18 19 20 21 22 23 24 25 26 27 28 29 30 31
July	8 9 10 11 12 13 14 15 16 17 18 19 20 21 22 23 24 25 26 27 28 29 30 31 1 2 3 4 5 6 7

Nov	1 2 3 4 5 6 7 8 9 10 11 12 13 14 15 16 17 18 19 20 21 22 23 24 25 26 27 28 29 30
Aug	8 9 10 11 12 13 14 15 16 17 18 19 20 21 22 23 24 25 26 27 28 29 30 31 1 2 3 4 5 6

Dec	1 2 3 4 5 6 7 8 9 10 11 12 13 14 15 16 17 18 19 20 21 22 23 24 25 26 27 28 29 30 31
Sept	7 8 9 10 11 12 13 14 15 16 17 18 19 20 21 22 23 24 25 26 27 28 29 30 1 2 3 4 5 6 7

Health and Diet

Feelings and hormones 22
Understanding how hormonal changes affect you emotionally

Health safeguards 24
Measures to take to preserve your well being while
you are pregnant

Physical changes 26
How pregnancy affects your body

Eating a healthy diet 28
Keeping at optimum health during pregnancy, including how to
plan a balanced diet

Essential nutrients 30
What to eat to stay healthy while you are pregnant

Morning sickness 32
How to cope with nausea and vomiting in the first three
to four months of pregnancy

Minor discomforts 34
Physical discomforts and conditions: what they are and
what to do

Getting bigger 38
Staying comfortable with your increased size: what to wear,
what to buy, and how to lie down

Traveling 40
Taking precautions when you travel and tips on what
to take with you

Reminders 42
Checklist of health tips for before, during, and
after pregnancy

HEALTH AND DIET

Taking care of yourself from the very first weeks of pregnancy is the most important thing you can do for the health of your baby. If you were planning to get pregnant, you may already have made some changes to your lifestyle. If you haven't, start taking extra care of your health from today.

2

You will find that your body is making its own changes. You will experience some emotional highs and lows and some physical discomforts as your body adjusts to its changing hormone levels. Ways are suggested to help you cope with these.

The most important thing is that you have a happy and relaxed pregnancy, without worrying too much. Knowing that you have taken sensible precautions to keep yourself in good health is the first step toward this.

FEELINGS AND HORMONES

Pregnancy is a time of both physical and emotional changes. Some women love being pregnant; others can't wait to get it over with. If this is your first baby, the emotional and physical impact that pregnancy has on your body may be alarming at first. Knowing why these changes are taking place and what to expect can help you to understand what's happening to your body and what you can do to help yourself.

FEELINGS AND EMOTIONS

However much you wanted a baby, now that you know you are pregnant, you are probably experiencing a mixture of conflicting emotions ranging from elation to apprehension. You may feel thrilled about being pregnant one day, doubtful about it the next. You may be excited about becoming a mother but worried about how you will cope, or you may burst into tears at the slightest provocation. These emotional highs and lows are perfectly natural, so don't feel guilty about them – many are triggered by an increase in hormones.

In addition to mood swings, rising hormone levels mean you may also experience a number of physical changes. How to cope with these is discussed on pp. 26–27. Once your hormones have stabilized, they may also help you to experience a sense of well-being and calmness. In fact, many pregnant women say they have never looked or felt better.

WHAT YOU CAN DO ABOUT NEGATIVE FEELINGS

■ Discuss how you feel with your husband, or with friends or relatives.

■ Have a good cry if you want to.

■ If you are worried about how your life will change, think of the positive benefits that having a child will bring. Acknowledging to yourself that your life will change once you have a child also means that you are being realistic: if you imagine that your life will continue as before, you are deceiving yourself.

■ Read up on pregnancy and parenting, and join a prenatal class so that you are well informed.

■ Things seem worse if you are tired or run down. Keep healthy by getting plenty of exercise, relaxing regularly, and eating a balanced diet (see pp. 28–29).

■ If you are seriously depressed or have a lot of worries that you feel you can't solve alone, seek professional help.

HORMONES

These are chemical substances that are produced by the endocrine glands and released into the bloodstream, where they are carried to different parts of the body. Hormones play a vital part in pregnancy, when their output is greater than at any other time of your life.

THE MAIN PREGNANCY HORMONES

Human chorionic gonadotrophin (HCG)	When a fertilized egg embeds in the wall of the uterus, HCG is produced and prevents menstruation. It also causes the body to produce more progesterone. Rising levels of HCG during the first three months are thought to be responsible for morning sickness.
Estrogen and progesterone	These are important in all aspects of pregnancy and control most of the changes that take place. For example, progesterone prepares the lining of the uterus to receive the fertilized egg, stimulates the growth of body tissue and fat, and gives you a sense of calmness. Together estrogen and progesterone stimulate the growth of the milk ducts in the breast, making the breasts swell and the areolae (the area around the nipples) enlarge and darken.
Relaxin	This softens the cervix and relaxes the pelvic muscles and ligaments in preparation for birth.
Oxytocin	This stimulates the uterus to contract and help push out the baby, and after birth it helps the uterus to shrink back to its normal size. It is also responsible for stimulating milk production during breastfeeding.
Prostaglandins	These are local hormone-type substances that are present in many tissues in the body. They stimulate the uterus to contract, which is why suppositories or gel containing prostaglandins may be inserted into the vagina to stimulate labor.
Cortisone	The levels of this hormone increase during pregnancy, which is part of the reason that allergic conditions such as asthma and eczema improve at this time.
Adrenaline, noradrenaline and endorphins	These hormones are responsible for increasing the heart rate and also have important effects on mood. Endorphins effect our sense of wellbeing and are the body's natural painkillers. The levels of endorphins in the body increase throughout pregnancy and peak during labor.
Prolactin and Human Placental Lactogen (HPL)	These are both milk-making hormones. They are secreted during pregnancy, but estrogen and progesterone delay milk production. Once the baby is delivered, estrogen and progesterone levels fall and milk is produced.

2

HEALTH SAFEGUARDS

2

During pregnancy, your natural immunity to infection may be lowered. Some infections that are usually harmless may be harmful to your baby's health and development during pregnancy. Although these infections are usually rare, it is wise to take extra precautions to avoid them or protect yourself against them. Some workplaces or occupations may also be harmful during pregnancy.

FOOD SAFETY

■ Avoid raw and undercooked meat and poultry. Be extra careful to wash cutting boards, plates, and utensils used for raw meat and poultry thoroughly. Wash your hands carefully after handling these foods.

■ Avoid any products that may contain uncooked meat or fish, such as pâté or sushi.

■ Avoid raw eggs and foods containing undercooked egg, such as mayonnaise.

■ Refrigerate all cooked and chilled food and dairy products.

■ Heat ready-made meals and ready-to-eat poultry until they are "piping hot" rather than eating them cold or lukewarm.

■ Do not drink unpasteurized cows', goats', or sheep's milk.

■ Avoid soft cheeses with white skin, such as Camembert and Brie, and the blue-veined varieties such as Stilton, Danish blue, Dolcelatte, and Gorgonzola. Other soft cheeses, such as cream cheese and cottage cheese, are safe.

■ Avoid soft-whip ice cream.

■ Wash all fresh fruits, vegetables, and salad foods thoroughly.

■ Discard any moldy foods and sprouting potatoes.

TAKING MEDICINE DURING PREGNANCY

If you are pregnant you should not take any medication without checking with your doctor first. But don't stop taking any prescribed medicines without checking with your doctor, as a lack of treatment could be more harmful than the drug. Common antibiotics such as penicillin are safe but tetracyclines can cause bone deformities and staining of the teeth. Some antibacterial drugs (Sulfonamides) should not be used in late pregnancy and some over-the-counter painkillers, cough and cold remedies, antacids or iron tablets, as well as antihistamines, should also be checked with your doctor. Excessive amounts of vitamins and many herbal remedies can also be dangerous.

COPING AT WORK

It is often during the first three months of pregnancy, when you may be battling morning sickness or tiredness, that you will find it difficult to work normally. If possible, arrange to arrive later and leave earlier. If medical problems such as high blood pressure occur, you may be advised to stop working; otherwise, you can continue to work until 28 weeks or longer. But don't push yourself to the limit by rushing around shopping on your lunch break or doing other extra activities. Give yourself plenty of rest breaks where possible, and make sure that you eat a nutritious lunch. You should also keep your legs raised when sitting at a desk. If you have to stand for long periods, wear support pantyhose and vary your position frequently. You should always avoid smoke-filled rooms.

2

AVOIDING INFECTIONS

Listeriosis	If contacted during pregnancy, listeriosis can result in miscarriage, stillbirth, or severe illness in a newborn baby. High levels of listeria bacteria have been found in some foods, such as soft cheeses, and pâté, and in small amounts in some frozen ready-made meals and ready-to-eat poultry.
Salmonella	This bacteria can cause severe food poisoning, and babies may be affected by their mother's high temperature. Salmonella is most frequently found in eggs, poultry, and raw meat.
Toxoplasmosis	The toxoplasma parasite can be caught from raw or undercooked meat, cat feces, and infected soil. It causes influenza-like symptoms in a healthy adult; but if caught during pregnancy, it may affect the unborn child. If you have already had this infection, you will be immune and you can establish this with a blood test. If you are not immune, avoid handling cat litter; if you must change the tray, wear gloves, discarding the gloves and washing your hands afterward. Wash your hands after handling cats and kittens; and wear gloves when gardening, and wash your hands afterward.
Chlamydiosis	Chlamydiosis is a rare disease that may cause pregnant women to miscarry. To avoid infection, do not have contact with sheep during lambing, with milking ewes that have recently given birth, with the afterbirth, or with newborn lambs.

PHYSICAL CHANGES

You will start noticing changes in your body almost as soon as you know you are pregnant. Hormonal activity increases (see pp. 22–23) as your body naturally prepares itself to nurture you and your baby through the next nine months.

BREAST CHANGES

Breast changes start early in pregnancy, and by 6–8 weeks your breasts will be noticeably larger. Your nipples and areolae (the circles of darker skin around the nipples) will darken, and the veins close to the surface may become larger. Increased progesterone and estrogen may make your breasts feel firm and tender, and you may feel some tingling.

By about 12–14 weeks, your breasts may start to produce colostrum, the milklike substance that will feed your baby for the first few days.

As your breasts grow, you should wear a good support bra with wide straps. It's better to be measured and fitted properly in the last few months. Use breast pads to catch colostrum leaks.

BREATHLESSNESS

As your baby grows and takes up more space, you may become breathless because your lungs do not have as much room to expand. Once your baby's head is engaged (see p. 72), you should feel more comfortable again.

To alleviate the problem, sit and stand as straight as possible and sleep propped up in bed.

SKIN CHANGES

The different amounts of hormones may cause some skin changes. These include brown uneven patches on the face (called chloasma); streaks or lines on the breasts, abdomen, and thighs (stretch marks); and a dark line from the top to the bottom of the abdomen. Dark lines or patches become worse in the sun, but disappear after pregnancy. Stretch marks fade to a silvery appearance, but never disappear completely. Most health professionals agree that these marks cannot be prevented by creams, but you may enjoy massaging moisturizer or oil into your skin.

WEIGHT GAIN

The amount of weight women gain during pregnancy varies, but most gain about 22–35 pounds (10–16.5kg). Although you will start to gain weight from the beginning of pregnancy, most of this weight accumulates in the second half. Aim for a moderate, steady weight gain – being seriously underweight or overweight may lead to complications during pregnancy or labor.

COMMON CHANGES DURING PREGNANCY

Vaginal discharge is likely to increase in pregnancy. See your doctor if it is smelly, itchy, or makes you sore.	■ Wear cotton underwear and panty liners.
Nails may grow faster than usual and become brittle.	■ Use a good nail-conditioning cream. ■ Treat yourself to a professional manicure.
Hair quality and texture often improve during pregnancy, but this is unpredictable.	■ Avoid permanents and chemical colorants.
Tiredness is common during pregnancy, especially during the first three and last three months.	■ Don't overdo things; rest when you can, but also try to get gentle exercise. ■ Eat a well-balanced diet. ■ Accept offers of help. ■ See your doctor if you feel excessively tired to rule out the possibility of anemia or an underactive thyroid.
Food aversions and cravings for strange or specific foods are common in pregnancy.	■ Don't worry, as long as your overall diet remains healthy – no single food is vital for health. ■ If you develop an aversion to one food out of a food group (see pp. 28–29), choose a substitute. ■ If you have cravings for nonfoods such as soil or laundry starch, see your doctor. Known as pica, these cravings may indicate a nutritional deficiency such as iron.
The need to **urinate frequently** is common during early and in late pregnancy when the uterus puts pressure on the bladder.	■ Avoid tea and coffee, which are diuretics. ■ Try to empty your bladder as soon as the urge occurs. ■ If you have pain or a burning sensation when passing urine, see your doctor in case you have an infection. ■ Minimize spicy foods and avoid carbonated beverages.

2

EATING A HEALTHY DIET

2

Eating a well-balanced diet during pregnancy should be a pleasure, not a worry. What you eat will become your baby's nourishment, so you need to make sure you are choosing foods that will build up enough stores of the necessary nutrients from day one of your pregnancy. A healthy diet will help you keep fit and healthy to meet the demands of pregnancy and labor, and help your body to prepare for breastfeeding your baby if you choose to do so.

UNDERSTANDING THE FOOD GROUPS

No single type of food is essential for health, and no single food can supply all the nutrients your body needs. A well-balanced diet is one that contains an adequate amount of carbohydrate, protein, fat, vitamins, and minerals. These can all be found in the six main food groups, which each have a range of recommended daily servings. If you select a variety of foods and the recommended number of servings from each of these groups, preferably on a daily basis, you are likely to be eating a healthy and balanced diet. If you dislike one type of food from a group – or develop an aversion to it during pregnancy – don't worry, there are always other healthy options to choose from.

CALORIES AND ENERGY

Although you need more energy than usual during pregnancy, your levels of physical activity and your metabolic rate slow down. This compensates for your increased needs. On average, you need to take in only 200–300 more calories a day than were necessary to maintain your prepregnancy weight, and this is for the final three months only. If you were underweight at the start of your pregnancy, you may need more calories.

All foods contain calories. But some, such as sugar, fat, and refined foods, are high in calories but low in nutrients. Others, such as grain products or fruit, have relatively few calories, but many nutrients – most of your calories should come from these foods. Base most of your meals around the carbohydrate group at the bottom of the food pyramid shown opposite. These foods are filling without being fattening, contain other nutrients in addition to carbohydrates, and are usually cheap.

To make up the extra calories, you can have nourishing snacks between meals. For ideas for healthy snacks, see p.31.

SPECIAL DIETS

If you follow a vegetarian or vegan (strict vegetarian) diet, discuss this with your doctor, nutritionist, or dietitian as soon as you know you are pregnant, as you may need vitamin and mineral supplements.

THIS FOOD PYRAMID SHOWS THE SIX MAIN GROUPS INTO WHICH FOODS ARE DIVIDED. USE THE SHAPE OF THE PYRAMID AS A GUIDELINE — EAT LESS OF THE FOODS AT THE TOP AND MORE OF THOSE AT THE BASE.

2

FATS, SUGAR, SALT, AND ALCOHOL

Eat sparingly since these contain few nutrients.

MEAT, POULTRY, FISH, BEANS, AND NUTS

Provide: Protein, vitamins A and B, fiber (nuts and beans), iron, and zinc. Servings needed: 2–3 daily (1 serving is 2–3 oz/50–70 g meat or fish, 2 eggs, 2 tbsp peanut butter, ½ cup cooked beans).

DAIRY PRODUCTS

PROVIDE: Calcium, protein, vitamin A (whole milk products), zinc, magnesium, and iodine. Servings needed: 2–3 daily. (1 serving is 1½ oz/ 40 g of cheese, 6 oz/ 175 ml milk or yogurt, ½ cup cottage cheese).

VEGETABLES

Provide: Fiber, vitamins A and C, folic acid, potassium, and iron. Servings needed: 3–5 or more daily. Select one serving from dark yellow or green leafy vegetables for Vitamin A. (1 serving is 1 cup of leafy greens, ½ cup cooked carrots or squash, 6 oz/175 ml of juice).

FRUITS

Provide: Fiber, vitamin C, and potassium. Servings needed: 2–4 or more daily. Select one serving from citrus fruits, tomatoes, or other fruits rich in vitamin C. (1 serving is 1 medium-sized apple, pear, or orange, 3 oz/90 ml of fruit juice).

BREAD, CEREAL, PASTA, AND RICE

Provide: Protein, fiber, vitamins, and minerals.
Foods that contain plenty of fiber include whole-wheat bread, baked potatoes, and wheat or oat bran breakfast cereals. Breakfast cereals are also usually fortified with vitamins and iron.
Servings needed: 6–11 daily. (1 serving is 1 slice of bread, ½ English muffin or small bagel, 1oz/30 g of cereal, ½ cup cooked rice or pasta).

ESSENTIAL NUTRIENTS

The following lists should help you change your eating habits and find the nutrients you need in familiar, everyday foods.

NUTRIENT	NEEDED FOR	GOOD SOURCES
Fiber	Helps prevent constipation and hemorrhoids. Too much can interfere with the absorption of iron and calcium.	Whole-wheat bread and pasta, some breakfast cereals, potatoes, fruit, vegetables, beans, and legumes.
Calcium	Muscle function, correct functioning of the immune system, and building bones and teeth.	Dairy products, darkgreen leafy vegetables, eggs, and fish. You need at least 1200mg a day.
Zinc	Growth and development.	Meat, dairy products, oysters, whole-wheat bread, cereals, beans, and nuts.
Iron	The formation of red blood cells, which carry oxygen to the tissues and fetus. Deficiency leads to anemia, which causes tiredness and shortness of breath.	Red meat, oily fish (such as canned sardines), fortified breakfast cereals, beans and legumes, pumpkin, dried apricots, and leafy green vegetables. Check with your doctor before taking an iron supplement: too much iron can be toxic. Keep iron tablets out of the reach of children.
Vitamins	General good health.	A balanced diet will usually provide all you need, but you should take a folic acid supplement (see p. 11) in the first 12 weeks of pregnancy. Prenatal vitamins are often recommended. An excess of Vitamin A may damage your baby.

2

CHANGING YOUR EATING HABITS

If you already have healthy eating habits, only small adjustments need be made to make sure you are getting adequate nutrients. If you are not used to a regular eating pattern, or eat a lot of junk food, try to improve your diet a little at a time.

■ Try to eat a variety of food from each of the main food groups every day.

■ Try to eat three regular meals a day. If you find this difficult, be flexible about the times and the amount. If you can't face breakfast, for example, have something substantial during the morning.

■ Have a minimum of six to eight beverages a day. Replace sugary or carbonated drinks and caffeine with water, low-fat milk, or herbal tea.

■ Meals don't have to be cooked if you don't have the time. A healthy snack (see below) can be as nourishing as a cooked meal.

■ To avoid eating too much saturated fat, limit full-fat products, and have low-fat substitutes instead.

■ Try eating dried fruits as a substitute for candy.

■ Limit salt in your cooking, avoid salty foods, and don't add extra salt to your plate.

■ Avoid processed foods such as pies, potato chips, cakes, and cookies, or candy.

■ Iron is absorbed better by the body if you eat iron-containing foods (such as red meat) with foods containing vitamin C (such as fruit or vegetables). Absorption of iron is reduced by drinking tea or coffee with a meal.

Healthy snacks

When you feel hungry and don't have time for a meal, try to avoid eating processed or refined foods. Instead, eat a snack that contains nutrients, rather than food with empty calories, such as:

■ A sandwich with a filling such as cheese, oily fish, hard-cooked egg, cooked meat and lettuce, banana and peanut butter

■ Whole-wheat toast with a topping such as cream cheese, cottage cheese, peanut butter, or hummus

■ Fresh or dried fruit

■ Raw vegetables with cheese dip or hummus

■ Low-sugar, low-fat yogurt with added fresh or canned fruit

■ Pizza with salad

■ A baked potato with grated cheese or natural yogurt

■ Crackers with hard cheese

■ A glass of low-fat milk and slice of fruit or carrot cake

■ Cheese cubes and walnuts

■ Whole-wheat breakfast cereal with added fruit

MORNING SICKNESS

Nausea and vomiting during the first three to four months of pregnancy is usually known as morning sickness. They can, however, happen at any time of the day and may vary from a slight feeling of nausea to actual vomiting. For some women it is the worst aspect of their pregnancy, but not all women suffer from it, and those who do can usually expect it to disappear by 12 to 14 weeks.

CAUSES

Morning sickness is thought to be caused by the hormone HCG, which rises during the first three months of pregnancy (see p. 23). HCG levels fall as the pregnancy progresses, and the sickness usually lessens. For a minority of women, however, feeling sick lasts throughout pregnancy.

Other trigger factors may be stress, strong smells, prenatal vitamins, iron tablets taken in the first three months of pregnancy, indigestion, and seeing or smelling food to which you are averse.

If you are excessively sick or your sickness persists after 16 weeks, consult your doctor.

HELPFUL THERAPIES

Some women have found that wearing wrist bands, designed to combat seasickness, are effective against morning sickness. Certain nutrients are also helpful: Ginger – tea or crystallized – may help, as can taking supplements of vitamin B6. If these remedies do not help, contact your doctor for advice.

Warning!
Severe or excessive vomiting during pregnancy, when a woman is unable to keep any food down and loses weight, is known as *hyperemesis gravidarum*. It occurs in about one in 200 pregnancies and must be treated by a doctor. Treatment for *hyperemesis gravidarum* is usually fast and effective, and the mother and baby are unlikely to suffer any lasting effects. In rare cases, admission to a hospital may be necessary.

WHAT YOU CAN DO

There are many simple remedies to help you cope with morning sickness. Try some of the suggestions below to see what works for you. If you do vomit, brush your teeth afterward to help prevent dental decay since vomit contains acid that attacks teeth.

■ Give yourself extra time to get somewhere without rushing.

■ Eat any food you like as soon as you're hungry.

■ Eat whatever will stay down.

■ Eat small snacks of carbohydrate foods such as toast, fruit, dry crackers, or plain cooked potato, little and often.

■ Avoid fatty foods and foods to which you have an aversion, and don't cook foods with strong smells.

■ Try eating foods high in vitamin B6: These include bananas, tuna, potatoes, wheat bran, raisins, and sesame seeds.

■ Try sucking mints, hard or ginger candy; or chew peppermint-flavored chewing gum.

■ Avoid medication unless prescribed.

■ If citrus juices or water upset you, try "defizzed" sodas (such as ginger ale or cola), carbonated drinks (such as spring water) or herbal teas, including peppermint and camomile.

■ Before you get out of bed in the morning, have a beverage and eat some dry, high-carbohydrate food such as a cookie or a piece of toast. Stay in bed for 20 minutes or so to give it time to digest.

■ Rise slowly and sit on the edge of the bed for a couple of minutes before standing up.

2

MINOR DISCOMFORTS

Most pregnant women experience minor discomforts or conditions at some stage of their pregnancy. Attention to overall health and fitness can minimize the impact of many of them, although few women escape them completely. Occasionally a symptom may be a sign of a more serious problem, so you should always consult your doctor if you are concerned about your health, or if a problem does not clear up after trying the simple self-help measures.

ACHES AND PAINS

These are common mainly because of the effect of hormones loosening the joints, and the ligaments being stretched and strained by your growing baby. Rib pain is caused by the growing uterus pushing the ribs up.

To relieve rib pain, stretch both arms above your head.

BACKACHE

Backache can occur at any stage, but may be especially troublesome during the last few weeks. It is usually due to the hormones loosening the pelvic joints and ligaments to prepare the body for labor, combined with strain on your back muscles as your growing baby alters your balance. Check severe backache with your doctor. Occasionally, it may be due to a kidney infection.

To prevent backache, always squat or bend from your knees to pick things up and avoid lifting heavy objects. When sitting, support the hollow of your back with a pillow and when standing, pay attention to your posture and stand "tall." You should also wear low-heeled shoes. Check that your bed is giving adequate support, and is neither too soft nor too hard.

If you are suffering from backache, apply heat or cold to the affected area and have plenty of rest; have a massage, or ask your doctor or physical therapist about special back exercises.

VARICOSE VEINS

These are due to increased weight, pressure from the enlarging uterus, and the effects of hormones, and although they are not serious they may cause aching or sore legs. To help avoid them, don't stand for long periods, and sit with your feet up whenever possible. Support hose may also be helpful; try showering at night and putting on the support hose before you get out of bed in the morning. Varicose veins of the vulva are also common. If you suffer from these, raise the foot of the bed slightly to take the pressure off your genitals.

2

SWOLLEN FEET AND ANKLES

Edema, or swelling of the feet and ankles, may occur because fluid is retained more easily in pregnancy, particularly at the end of the day and in hot weather. To alleviate the swelling, try foot circles (p. 54), avoid standing or sitting for long periods, wear support hose and comfortable shoes, and rest with your legs up whenever possible Always mention any swelling in the hands and face to your doctor – this could be a sign of preeclampsia.

ITCHING

Itching caused by the stretched abdominal skin is common in late pregnancy. Apply a cream for dry skin or calamine lotion and avoid using soap. Wear light clothes in natural fabrics, choosing several layers in cold weather, and avoid anything stretchy like lycra next to your abdomen. In rare cases, it may be caused by a liver problem, so consult your doctor if itching is excessive or if your skin looks yellow.

OTHER CONDITIONS

There are a number of other conditions you may become concerned about as your pregnancy progresses. Many of these are easily explained and quickly relieved. However, if a problem persists, see your doctor.

CONDITION	WHAT TO DO
Faintness can occur if your blood pressure drops due to a sudden change of position, or drop in blood sugar level. You may also feel faint when lying on your back in late pregnancy.	■ Get up slowly after sitting or lying down, loosen any tight clothing, and place a cool, damp cloth on your forehead. ■ Avoid lying on your back in late pregnancy. ■ Avoid long periods without food, as this can cause a drop in blood sugar. ■ Avoid sugary food. Have a healthy snack such as a sandwich or a banana (see p. 31).
Nosebleeds occur because there is an increased supply of blood to the nose during pregnancy.	■ Gently squeeze your nostrils together, just below the bony bridge of the nose, for at least 5–10 minutes. ■ If your nasal passages are dry, gently apply petroleum jelly on a cotton swab. ■ If bleeding is persistent, consult your doctor.
Sinuses are more sensitive and can swell, causing headaches and nasal congestion.	■ Try a steam inhalation to help relieve congestion, adding one or two drops of eucalyptus or peppermint oil.
Indigestion and heartburn are mainly due to hormones relaxing the stomach muscles. These are often worse at night or when lying down.	■ Try to identify which foods are causing the problem and avoid them. ■ Eat small but frequent meals. ■ Avoid highly spiced, very cold, or fried foods. ■ Sit up straight while eating and sleep propped up. ■ Ask your doctor about antacids.
Tingling and numbness in the hands is usually due to pressure on nerves.	■ Change your position or raise your hands above your head. ■ Try hanging a numbed hand over the side of the bed or shaking it vigorously.
Headaches may occur more often than usual during pregnancy, probably due to hormonal factors.	■ Take a walk. ■ Try relaxation techniques (see pp. 58-61). ■ If necessary, ask your doctor to recommend a safe painkiller. If your headaches are severe or accompanied by vomiting or edema, contact your doctor.

2

CONDITION	WHAT TO DO
Stress incontinence is leakage of urine when you laugh, cough, or sneeze. It is caused by weak pelvic floor muscles. It may occur during the last months of pregnancy or following delivery.	■ Do pelvic floor exercises (see p. 55). ■ Wear a sanitary pad or panty liner if necessary. ■ Urinate as soon as you feel the urge. ■ Try to empty your bladder completely: to do this, sit forward on the toilet. ■ Avoid bladder irritants, such as carbonated beverages, coffee, tea, and spicy foods.
Muscle cramps are probably due to chemical and hormonal changes in the body.	■ Avoid pointing your toes when you stretch your legs since this can trigger cramps. ■ Gently massaging your calf muscles in the bathtub before bedtime may help cramps at night. ■ If a spasm occurs, pull your feet toward your face with your leg straight. ■ Massage your legs.
Pelvic pain is due to the loosening and stretching of the ligaments.	■ Lie down. ■ Take a warm bath. ■ Massage the area. ■ Try some gentle exercises (see pp. 54-55). ■ Consult your doctor about any severe pelvic or abdominal pain. If pelvic pains are severe, you may need complete rest.
Constipation is common and probably due to the effect of the hormone progesterone. During later months, pressure from the enlarged uterus on the bowels can make the problem worse.	■ Make sure your diet contains plenty of high-fiber foods (see p. 30). ■ Drink plenty of fluids (especially water and fruit juices). ■ Exercise daily: a brisk walk, plus pelvic floor and other safe pregnancy exercises, will help. ■ If the problem persists, ask your doctor to recommend a stool softener. Avoid using laxatives.
Hemorrhoids are swollen veins in and around the rectum and are common in pregnancy. Symptoms include: itching, soreness, pain with bowel movement, and bleeding. They are worsened by constipation.	■ Avoid constipation (see above). ■ Stop smoking. ■ Exercise regularly and practice relaxation. ■ Use warm water or moist tissues instead of paper to wipe yourself. ■ Apply a soft cold compress of witch hazel, Epsom salts, or an ice pack. ■ Try a hemorrhoid cream or suppository. ■ Always have bleeding from the rectum checked by your doctor.

2

GETTING BIGGER

A s your body continues to grow, being comfortable can sometimes pose problems. Some of your clothes and shoes will start to feel tight and you may wonder what to wear. You may also have difficulty finding a comfortable sleeping position. But there are several measures you can take to help you stay comfortable and to continue looking good throughout pregnancy.

2

WHAT TO WEAR

■ Up to around five months you probably won't need to buy any special clothes for your pregnancy. Many of your normal clothes will be wearable if they are loose or have elasticized waists.

■ Wear loose cotton tops, such as baggy T-shirts and sweaters, skirts with elasticized waists, and loose-fitting dresses or borrow your spouse's shirts, sweaters, and shorts, which are cut big and baggy.

■ Tight clothing will not harm your baby, but constricted clothing around the waist will be uncomfortable for you, and as your size increases, may restrict your breathing and make you feel faint. Avoid, too, clothes that restrict the blood flow to your legs, such as kneesocks or tight underwear.

■ You will tend to feel the heat more than usual, so lightweight loose-fitting clothes made of cotton or other natural materials are best. If it is cold, wear several layers.

■ Shoes with a low heel are better for your back and for your overall posture than totally flat shoes or high-heeled shoes, which can be dangerous. After five or six months, you may find that you need a wider shoe or shoes half a size bigger. Shoes made of natural material such as leather or canvas allow your feet to breathe.

■ Replace elastic in the waist of comfortable skirts or sweatpants with a drawstring that can be loosened as your waist expands.

■ It is worth asking friends who have had babies if they have any hand-me-downs. (Purchases like a maternity jacket or a party dress are easy to pass on.)

WHAT TO BUY

■ 2–3 well-fitting support bras/nursing bras if you are going to breastfeed. Some maternity shops measure you for these – it is difficult to judge for yourself how big you might get when your milk comes in.

■ 1–2 pairs of shoes ½-size larger or wider (especially if the last months of your pregnancy are in summer).

■ 2–3 front-opening nightgowns/pairs of pajamas if you are going to breastfeed (you will need these in the hospital).

■ Buy extra-large pantyhose or support hose instead of the more expensive maternity tights.

■ Bikini-style panties that can be worn under your bump, or large, stretchy ones that you can pull up over it are more comfortable than regular ones. Cotton panties or at least panties with a cotton crotch are best.

■ Buy clothes such as dresses and bras with a front opening for breastfeeding, so that you can get some wear out of them after pregnancy.

■ Several mail-order companies specialize in maternity wear and offer good value for money because everything is coordinated: a pair of slacks or leggings, skirt, dress, and a couple of T-shirts, for example, offers enormous scope for mixing and matching.

2

GETTING YOUR REST

During the last months of pregnancy, you may find sleeping more difficult because comfortable positions can be harder to find. In addition, the extra weight you are carrying around may also make you feel very tired. To help sleeplessness and exhaustion:

■ Try drinking a glass of warm milk at bedtime, or having a warm bath with a few drops of lavender oil added, to help you relax.

■ Take short naps or rest during the day.

■ Practice your relaxation techniques.

■ Try lying on your side with one leg bent and a pillow supporting your knee. You could also place a pillow under your abdomen if this is more comfortable.

TRAVELING

It is generally safe to travel during pregnancy, but sometimes it can be quite exhausting. If you are going to travel long distances, plan your journey carefully. In the first three months (first trimester), you may suffer from nausea or vomiting, and throughout pregnancy, the need to urinate frequently can be a problem on long journeys.

The most comfortable time for long-distance travel is during the second three months (second trimester). By this time your body will have adjusted to pregnancy, and you will feel at your fittest and best. Morning sickness is usually no longer a problem, and you will probably have the stamina to sit for long periods of time.

WHAT TO TAKE

Your maternity record card if you plan to be away for more than a day, in case you need to see a doctor in an emergency

Antibacterial or medicated hand wipes in case you cannot wash your hands

Some light but healthy snacks and fluids, so that food and drink is readily available if you need it (see p.31).

Travel bands in case of nausea

Light sanitary pads or panty liners if you have a heavy vaginal discharge or stress incontinence

DRIVING

When you travel by car, it is essential to wear a correctly fitted seat belt. A seat belt worn high across the abdomen can be dangerous to you and your baby in the event of an accident. The safest way to wear a seat belt is with the shoulder harness between the breasts and the lap belt across the thighs so that it fits under the abdomen. Try to avoid driving during rush hour so that you are not breathing heavy fumes. On long trips, try to take short stops every hour or two, and walk around to stretch your legs. In the second or third trimester, do not undertake anything longer than a three-hour drive if you are driving alone.

2

AIR TRAVEL

If you plan to travel late in your pregnancy, check with your doctor about the chance of premature labor. Most airlines limit their flights to women no closer than four weeks from their due date. The metal detectors used for airline security checks are not harmful to the fetus. Feet can swell when traveling by air even if you are not pregnant, so make extra sure your shoes are not too tight. Walk around and stretch frequently.

GENERAL TIPS

- Try to divide up long journeys into shorter, manageable sections.
- Wear loose, comfortable clothes that do not restrict you.
- Remember to empty your bladder frequently.
- Do not take any motion-sickness pills without first checking with your doctor.
- If you plan to be away from home for some time, you may need to sign up temporarily with another doctor in your new area. Ask your doctor for a referral.
- If you are traveling abroad, ask your doctor what vaccinations are necessary, and whether these are safe to get during pregnancy. If possible, avoid visiting a country where you have a chance of contracting an infectious disease such as malaria or cholera.

REMINDERS

Being healthy before you conceive – and staying healthy during pregnancy – will give your baby the best possible start in life. Use this list as a reminder of what to do before and after conception to make sure you and your baby get all the nutrients you need, and avoid as many potential hazards as possible.

WHEN YOU ARE TRYING TO CONCEIVE

■ Take a daily folic acid supplement (at least 400 micrograms/0.4mg) in the three months before you plan to conceive and during the first 12 weeks of pregnancy.

■ Check whether you are immune to rubella (German measles).

■ Ask your doctor's advice on whether to seek genetic screening or other tests.

■ Cut out smoking and recreational drugs, and limit your alcohol intake.

WHEN YOU BECOME PREGNANT

■ Avoid alcohol.

■ Don't smoke and avoid smoky rooms.

■ If you need an X ray, make sure you tell the technician you are pregnant.

■ Don't take any unprescribed medicines, vitamin or mineral supplements, herbal remedies or herbal teas containing aloe, coltsfoot, heart's ease, licorice, nutmeg, pennyroyal, sassafras, and tansy.

■ Avoid contact with people suffering from infectious diseases.

■ Avoid contact with chemicals, lead paint, and other toxic materials; don't mix household cleaners containing ammonia with those containing chlorine.

■ Wear gloves when gardening; avoid changing cat litter and avoid contact with sheep and lambs during lambing season.

■ Eat a well-balanced diet. Take extra care when storing and preparing food.

■ Wash fruit and vegetables thoroughly, even those sold as "ready washed."

■ Avoid eating raw or lightly cooked eggs or food containing these products.

■ Don't eat liver or liver products, such as fresh pâté and liver sausage.

■ Don't take fish oil supplements.

■ Don't eat unripened cheeses such as Brie, Camembert, and blue-vein cheeses.

■ Don't eat food that has passed its sell-by date.

■ Reduce your intake of sugary carbonated drinks and caffeine.

■ Cook all foods until they are heated thoroughly.

■ Wear a correctly fitted seat belt when traveling by car.

■ Consult your doctor if you feel unwell, start bleeding after your pregnancy has been confirmed, suffer prolonged or severe pregnancy sickness, or are worried in any way.

Exercise and Relaxation

EXERCISE AND RELAXATION

Regular exercise and adequate rest combined with a well-balanced diet will help you maintain good health during your pregnancy. Exercise improves your circulation, makes you supple, gives you stamina, and improves muscle tone. Appropriate exercise before conception and during pregnancy will help to limit your weight gain, reduce backache, may minimize stretch marks, and lead to a quicker postpartum recovery. Improvements to your circulation will reduce or help to alleviate such common problems as varicose veins, constipation, and raised blood pressure. The exercises on the following pages will help you tone up before, during, and after pregnancy.

Stress and tension are bad for you and may also affect your baby. They cause headaches, tightening of the muscles, and backache. Exercise will help you to relax, but learning breathing and specific relaxation techniques will be invaluable in helping you breathe correctly and help control pain during labor and delivery.

3

GETTING FIT

Women who are fit tend to cope better with pregnancy and labor than those who are not. If you make exercise part of your life before you conceive, you are more likely to continue with it when you are pregnant. In the three months before conceiving, build regular exercise – at least three times a week – into your daily routine. Consult your doctor first if you have been ill or have a physical disability. If you are already pregnant, consult your doctor before taking up anything new.

WHAT KIND OF EXERCISE?

Remember, you are more likely to stick to a prepregnancy exercise program if you are doing something you enjoy.

■ Moderate exercise such as half an hour's brisk walking a day is beneficial: walk to work, or walk a couple of stops before taking the bus or train.

■ Take up a sport you enjoyed at school, or one you've always wanted to learn. Consider swimming, tennis, golf, or an aerobics, or stretch class.

■ Go for a bicycle ride (or try an exercise bike at a gym; if you like it, consider buying one or joining the gym).

■ Try gardening. Offer to take your neighbor's dog for a walk, or play ball with a friend's or neighbor's child.

■ Buy a jump rope and use it.

■ Join a dance class or put on a favorite record and dance around the room.

EXERCISING SAFELY

■ Check with your doctor before starting any exercise regime.

■ Take it easy to start with, and always warm up before you start and cool down when you have finished.

■ Don't exercise on a full or empty stomach: have a high carbohydrate snack, such as a banana or some rice cakes, about half an hour before you start.

■ Make sure your exercise teacher is qualified; ask to see credentials.

■ Always use the right kind of shoes and equipment; wear loose clothing.

■ Never push yourself to the limit. Stop if you feel breathless, exhausted, or are in pain.

■ If it's effective, exercise will make you sweat; be sure to drink plenty of fluids.

3

BASIC EXERCISE POSITION

Poor posture can lead to damaged muscles when you exercise. In addition, learning the "feel" of good posture now will pay dividends when you are pregnant, when your changing shape will throw your body out of alignment. When exercising, check that:

■ You are standing with your feet shoulder-width apart (unless suggested otherwise) and your toes pointing slightly outward.

■ Your stomach muscles are pulled in.

■ Your shoulders are relaxed and down.

■ Your knees are over your feet.

■ Your hips are square to the front and over your knees.

3

PREPREGNANCY EXERCISES FOR STAMINA

Aerobic exercise that increases your heart rate helps to build up stamina, improves your circulation, and increases your metabolic rate; it also makes you feel good. Some aerobic exercises also improve your overall strength. Good aerobic exercises include:

■ Brisk steady walking – at a rate of 5 MPH (8 km/h) – ideally including some hills.

■ Swimming: increase the strength of your arms by wearing webbed gloves to give resistance to the water. If you like swimming, you may also enjoy water aerobics.

■ Jogging: running at a rate of 6 MPH (9.5 km/h) is even better.

■ Low impact aerobic/step/keep fit classes. High-impact aerobics, which can injure your legs, should only be done if you are very fit, and not during pregnancy.

■ Bicycling: indoors or out; this also increases the strength of your legs.

■ Racquet sports such as tennis, racquetball, and squash.

■ Jumping rope: buy a proper rope; turning it should be effortless.

■ Rowing: this also increases strength in your arms and legs.

EXERCISE IN PREGNANCY

If your pregnancy is progressing normally and without any complications, moderate regular exercise is safe and beneficial to your health. It will improve your circulation, make your muscles stronger, and your joints more supple. Exercise can also lessen some of the discomforts of pregnancy such as constipation and fatigue, and help you relax. If you are physically fit, you are also likely to have an easier pregnancy, labor, and postpartum recovery.

GUIDELINES FOR EXERCISE DURING PREGNANCY

Most forms of exercise are safe to continue throughout pregnancy, but it is always worth checking with a physical therapist or your doctor. Always follow the basic guidelines for exercise on page 48. And, in addition, while you are pregnant, it is particularly important to:

- Avoid jarring and high impact motions. All your muscles are more vulnerable than normal during pregnancy and you risk tears or strains. Always check the surface on which you are working for this reason: it should have some give.
- If you attend exercise classes, make sure your teacher is qualified and knows you are pregnant.
- To avoid dehydration, drink small amounts often. Eat small, frequent, high-carbohydrate snacks, especially if you are suffering from heartburn.
- Don't exercise in very hot or humid weather or let yourself get too hot. In an effort to cool you down, your body diverts blood from the baby.
- Always wear a well-fitting support bra designed for exercise. Make sure your shoes are appropriate. Check with an instructor if you are in doubt.
- Monitor your pulse rate: it should not rise above 140 beats per minute.

3

Warning!

If you have a history of recurrent miscarriage or a complicated pregnancy, exercise should be particularly gentle and moderate. Some women may be advised by their doctor to rest and not to exercise at all.

Stop exercising if you experience any of these symptoms:

- vaginal bleeding
- leak or gush of amniotic fluid
- pain of any kind
- contractions or abdominal pain
- nausea, dizziness, or faintness
- shortness of breath
- palpitations or very rapid heartbeat

- any swelling or numbness
- pain in the legs
- difficulty in walking
- persistent headaches
- visual disturbances
- decreased fetal movements
- excessive tiredness

SPORTS IN PREGNANCY

Swimming and water exercise	Swimming is an excellent exercise for your body because it uses many different muscles while the water supports your weight. Women who swim several times a week usually have very strong abdominal muscles after the birth of their baby. You may also enjoy doing some water exercises as a safe way of maintaining or improving your flexibility in pregnancy.
Jogging or running	If you were used to running or jogging before you became pregnant, you can continue during pregnancy. Avoid marathon running or jogging more than 3 miles (5 km) a day. Don't become overheated or too tired, and drink plenty of fluids. Make extra sure, too, that you wear well-supporting cushioned shoes to prevent jarring, and if possible, jog on soft rather than hard surfaces. As your pregnancy progresses, you may find that jogging becomes more difficult.
Aerobic exercise	If you are used to going to aerobic classes, let the instructor know that you are pregnant. View aerobic exercise in pregnancy as maintaining your fitness, rather than improving it. Don't overexert yourself; work at a pace that allows you to hold a conversation without getting out of breath.
Bicycling	If you are comfortable doing so, there is no reason why you should not cycle during pregnancy. The main risk to the baby is from an accident that may cause a miscarriage or premature labor, and toward the end of pregnancy, your shape may make you less stable. Whenever possible, avoid main or busy roads because of the risk of traffic pollution.
Horseback riding	Many women go horseback riding while pregnant, however, a fall is dangerous, so check with your doctor.
Ice skating	Avoid jumping; otherwise, ice skating can be carried on in a modified form for as long as you can get your skates on!
Skiing	There is a risk of falling with force and harming your baby. Skiing while pregnant is not recommended.
Water sports	Water sports such as waterskiing, scuba diving, and platform diving are not recommended.

3

STRETCHING

Stretching during pregnancy is both an exercise and a way to relax. Simple stretches should also be used as warm-ups and for cooling down, before and after more vigorous exercise. Stretching can help relieve minor discomforts such as backache, and by toning up the muscles and opening up your pelvic area, it will help you to prepare for birth.

GENERAL GUIDELINES

Stretching is generally safe as long as you keep a few points in mind.

■ If you are not used to stretching, work up to it – five minutes a day is fine to start with.

■ Do not jump, bounce, or use jerky movements – move smoothly into position.

■ Breathe deeply as you stretch and relax into it.

■ Be aware that the hormone relaxin causes an increased range of movements during pregnancy. As the long-term effects of this are not known, use short stretches rather than progressively increasing your range of movements.

■ Holding a position for your usual length of time may become a strain; if it does, hold briefly and repeat several times.

■ Do not lie flat on your back to stretch from the middle of pregnancy, as the baby may press against a major blood vessel, making you feel faint.

■ Throughout all these movements, be aware of your breathing and never hold your breath.

ARM STRETCHING

This helps to lift your ribs off your expanding uterus.

1 Sit in a position that is comfortable: either cross-legged on the floor or against a wall with your legs straight out in front of you.

2 Place your hands on your shoulders, then lift both hands above your head.

3 Stretch one arm higher than the other, reaching for the ceiling. Relax and repeat with the other arm. Repeat the exercise ten times.

4 With both arms raised, swing them down to shoulder height, bring your hands back to touch your shoulders and raise your arms again. Repeat ten times.

SHOULDER STRETCH

This can relieve heartburn and tension in your shoulders.

1 Stand up straight. Raise your right arm above your hand and drop it down between your shoulder blades.

2 At the same time, bend your left elbow and reach behind with your left hand. Touch or interlock fingers, if you can. (If you can't reach your other hand, try holding a belt or tie between your hands.) Hold for a count of five, breathing normally.

3 Repeat, with your left hand placed over your shoulder.

4 You can increase this stretch by gently pressing down on your elbow.

3

THE CAT STRETCH

This eases tension in your back and shoulders.

1 Kneel on the floor. Bend forward from the hips with your head down. Slowly "walk" your hands forward so that your arms are extended in front of you. Without arching your back, hold for a count of five, breathing normally.

2 Slowly sink down toward your thighs so that your bottom rests on your heels. Repeat three or four times, then sit up slowly.

GENTLE EXERCISES

If you don't want to, or are unable to, do any sports, attend exercise classes, or actively exercise, there are still some gentle exercises you can do to keep fit, supple, and toned during pregnancy. Unless otherwise stated, these exercises can be done throughout your pregnancy, but as your baby grows, you will become more breathless; and particularly during the last two to three months your mobility and balance will change. Choose exercises that do not aggravate any of these conditions.

INNER THIGH STRETCH

Strong, supple thighs will help to keep you mobile and are essential if you want to deliver your baby in a standing or semisquatting position.

1 Sit on the floor with your back straight, legs as far apart as you can comfortably get them, and shoulders back.

2 Lean forward from the waist and gradually "walk" your hands out in front of you. When you feel mild tension in your inner thighs, hold for a count of five, then relax. Return to an upright position and repeat three times.

THIGH RAISES

This will also strengthen your thighs and improve your overall mobility.

1 Lie on your side with your lower leg slightly bent at the knee. Support your head on your elbow.

2 Gradually raise your upper leg. Keep it straight but do not lock your knee. When it is as high as is comfortable, hold for a count of five, then lower it. Repeat three times, then repeat on your other side.

SQUATTING

This exercises the pelvic muscles and strengthens the inner thighs. It is a good position to practice for labor, and to adopt when doing pelvic floor exercises. As you grow bigger or if you have difficulty in keeping your balance, support yourself by holding the seat of a chair or the edge of a bed.

1 Stand with your feet shoulder width apart. Bending down at your hips and knees, slowly ease yourself into a squatting position.

2 Keeping your back straight and your feet flat on the floor, hold for up to 30 seconds if you can.

3

INNER THIGH STRETCH

This stretches the inner thigh muscles and increases the mobility of your pelvis and hip joint.

1 Sit on the floor with your back straight. Bring the soles of your feet together and let your knees drop toward the ground.

2 Hold your ankles and relax your hips so that your knees are even closer to the floor. Hold for a few seconds, extending these for a few seconds longer as it gets easier. Try to do once or twice a day.

UPPER BODY STRETCH

1 Sit on the floor with your legs wide apart. Bend your left knee and tuck your left foot into your body. Touch your right foot with your right fingers.

2 Breathe in as you raise your left arm above your head and reach toward your right foot. When you feel mild tension in your side, hold for a count of five.

ABDOMINAL EXERCISES

During pregnancy, your abdominal muscles, which run from your breastbone down to your pubic bone, take most of the extra weight of the baby. If these are flabby, your back muscles have to work harder to protect your spine, which in turn can cause backache. Strong, well-toned abdominal muscles during pregnancy not only help to protect your back, but will also return to condition more quickly after the birth.

CURL-UPS (FOR THE FIRST 3 MONTHS ONLY)

These strengthen your abdominal muscles. Never do curl- or sit-ups with your legs straight during pregnancy.

1 Lie on your back with your knees bent and feet flat on the floor. Place your hands behind your head. Breathe in.

2 Breathe out as you pull in your stomach muscles and slowly lift your head, shoulders, and upper back off the floor. Hold for the count of two, then slowly lower yourself back on the floor. Repeat five to ten times.

3 If this is difficult, you may find it easier to rest your arms on your thigh and inhale. As you exhale, move your arms toward your knees, at the same time lifting your head and shoulders off the floor. Roll back slowly and repeat five to ten times.

KNEELING PELVIC TILT

1 Kneel on the floor with your hands directly under your hips, and your back flat on the floor.

2 Tighten your abdominal and buttock muscles, and breathing out, gently tilt your pelvis forward and hump up your back. Hold this position for a few seconds, then relax.

STANDING PELVIC TILT

This exercise, which helps you move your pelvis with ease, is a good preparation for labor. It also tones your abdominal muscles and is helpful if you suffer from backache. You can do this exercise in a kneeling, sitting, or standing position. You can also roll your hips in a gentle circular movement.

1 Stand with feet well apart and knees directly over ankles, and place one hand on your lower back, and another under your "bump."

2 Drawing in your abdominal and buttock muscles, gently rock your pelvis back and forth.

POSTURE DURING PREGNANCY

Poor posture during pregnancy – when your behind sticks out and your back hollows – can lead to low backache and unnecessary strain on your body. Poor posture is aggravated by wearing high-heeled shoes, and by carrying a bag over the same shoulder, or a child on the same hip, all the time. A bra that offers inadequate support may make you round your shoulders as your breasts become heavier. Be fitted for a good bra.

Good posture involves using your abdominal and buttock muscles to support your baby. Stand with your feet evenly planted, about hip-width apart and in line with each other. Keep your knees loose and directly over your ankles. Let your shoulders drop down and your arms hang loosely from your sides

Visualize a string attached to the top of your head and pulling upward through your spine and neck so that your spine is straight and upright. Pull in your abdominal muscles so that your baby nestles toward your spine, rather than sitting out in front of you.

Keep remembering to check your posture and pull your abdominal muscles in.

3

Warning!

After every exercise session, or after exercises which involve lying on the floor, lie down and relax for a few minutes as shown on page 61. Then get up slowly, using your hands to push to a kneeling or sitting position first. If you lie on a bed, turn onto your side and keeping your legs together swing them over the side.

OTHER "EASY" EXERCISES

Even if you are not used to exercising, if your activity is restricted, or your work involves long periods of sitting, you still need to try to keep toned and supple. Remember to do the pelvic floor exercise daily (see right), which can be done at any time and any place. Also try some or all of the following other exercises – do whichever ones suit you. For example, if you cannot go for a walk, try walking or marching on the spot. Remember, though, that aerobic exercise does not have to involve vigorous exercise.

LOW-IMPACT AEROBICS

This builds up your stamina and includes brisk walking, marching on the spot, and swimming.

MARCHING ON THE SPOT

1 Stand in the correct posture for exercising (see p. 45). Start with brisk walking on the spot, lifting your knees and transfering your weight from foot to foot.

2 Increase your pace so that you are "marching." See how high you can lift your knees. Swing your arms freely. Raise your arms up and down, touching each shoulder. Cross them over so your right arm touches your left knee and vice versa.

3 Take two steps forward and clap your hands on the third. Repeat, walking backward.

FOOT AND ANKLE EXERCISES

These can reduce swelling and help circulation.

1 Circle each foot in turn five times in one direction and five in the other.

2 Practice drawing the whole alphabet with your feet, one foot at a time. Keep your legs still but move your ankles.

HEAD ROLLS

1 Gently let your head bend forward, stretching your neck, hold for a few seconds, and lift.

2 Turn it to one side, then face forward, bend head, lift. Repeat with other side in a continual flow. Do not let your head roll back.

SHOULDER ROLLS

1 To relieve tension and increase suppleness, slowly circle each shoulder backward several times in turn.

2 Lift both shoulders up, press them gently back, and pull them down.

3

PELVIC FLOOR EXERCISES

These are essential but simple and effective exercises which strengthen the muscles around the bladder and vagina, and can help to prevent or control stress incontinence before and after delivery. They should be practiced several times an hour throughout the day, and are easily done at any time, such as when you are on the telephone, standing, washing dishes, waiting for a bus, etc. To know you have located your muscles, try stopping the flow of urine when you go to the bathroom – but do this only to make sure you are practicing properly and not as a routine part of the exercise.

1 Sit, stand, or lie with legs slightly apart.

2 Close and draw up the sphincter muscles around your anal opening as if preventing gas or a bowel action. At the same time, draw in your vaginal muscles as if to grip a tampon or avoid passing urine.

3 Hold tight and count to four, breathing normally. Relax and repeat. Do these as often as possible every day.

AFTER THE BIRTH

During the first few days after birth, as well as facing all the excitement and demands of a newborn baby, you may be feeling sore and exhausted. Exercise is likely to be the last thing you feel like doing. But exercising to get your shape back is important and is most successful when it is progressive and gentle. Start right from the first day after birth, with breathing exercises, foot circles (see p. 54), and pelvic floor exercises (see pp. 55–57). Pelvic floor exercises are the most important you can do: practice as often as possible, but at least 30 times a day. They help to stop any urine from leaking, help stitches to heal, and ease perineal pain. They also tighten your vaginal muscles, which will make intercourse more pleasurable. From the third day after delivery, add pelvic tilts (see p. 52), leg slides, and the pelvic rock. These exercises can be done even if you have had a cesarean section.

BREATHING EXERCISES

This is a gentle way to strengthen your abdominal muscles. Do them three times before any other exercises.

1 Lie on your bed with your knees bent or sit fully supported in an armchair. Relax your shoulders, place your hands on your abdomen so that you can feel it rise, and breathe in slowly and deeply through your nose.

2 Breathe out slowly through your mouth, tightening your abdominal muscles as you do so.

PELVIC ROCK

1 Lie on your back on the bed or floor with your knees bent and feet flat.

2 Tighten your buttocks, tilt them up, and draw in your abdomen so that the small of your back rolls flat against the bed or floor. Hold, then relax.

LEG SLIDES

1 Lie flat on your back with your knees bent and feet resting on the bed. Breathing in, slide one leg from a bent to a straight position.

2 Breathing out, bend it back again. Repeat with the other leg.

HEAD LIFTS

After about a week, gently move on to more active abdominal exercises.

1 Lie on your back with your knees bent, feet flat on the floor, and arms by your side. Breathe in and relax your abdomen. Breathing out, lift your head off the floor. Hold for the count of two, then slowly lower your head back.

2 When you feel comfortable doing 10 head lifts, proceed to lifting your shoulders and upper back off the floor, too.

3

3 Once you feel comfortable doing shoulder lifts, proceed to full curl-ups (see p. 52).

CLOSING THE MUSCLE GAP

During pregnancy, strong abdominal muscles help to carry the extra weight of the baby and support your spine. But unless you were highly toned before you became pregnant, these muscles are likely to have stretched and may have parted by the time your baby is born. Depending on the size of the gap, and the amount of exercise you do, the muscles close together in the first few days or weeks after the birth.

To check for abdominal separation:

■ Lie on your back with your knees bent.

■ Put the fingers of one hand on your abdomen just below your navel and press in gently.

■ Slowly lift your head and shoulders and stretch your other hand forward. If you feel a gap or soft lump the width of a finger or more, the muscles have separated.

To close the gap:

■ Do head lifts (above).

If you can still feel the gap after six weeks, ask a physical therapist for specific exercises.

RELAXATION TECHNIQUES

R elaxing your body and mind during pregnancy gives those parts of your body that may ache, such as your back, abdomen, and legs, a chance to recuperate from the stress of carrying extra weight around and of holding your body upright. It helps to relieve stress, which may contribute to raised blood pressure, and helps to keep your brain active.

Some people find relaxing easier than others do. If the basic relaxation exercise on p.61 does not work for you, there are many other, more formal techniques which pregnant women have found useful. Some of these need to be taught; others can be practiced at home.

RELAXING

Relaxation techniques are simple, but you do have to find the time to practice them. You do not have to practice at the same time every day, but you may find it easier to keep a routine if you do make 15 to 20 minutes each day to relax. Perhaps you could get up slightly earlier each day, or make time when you get home from work, or right after you take a bath or shower. Total relaxation means not allowing troublesome or stimulating thoughts to disturb your peace. You may find some of these measure helpful:

- Choose a warm, quiet room. Close the curtains or blinds if activity outdoors will distract you.

- Wear loose clothes and sit in a comfortable position, with your back supported. Use as many pillows as you need to make you comfortable.

- Concentrate on your breathing; breathe slowly and evenly, using your abdominal muscles.

- Play some tranquil music or listen to some poetry, either on the radio or on a personal cassette or CD player.

- Think about what you enjoy doing, perhaps visualizing a slow, peaceful walk in beautiful surroundings, or along a beach.

- If you pray regularly, you may find that setting aside some time each day to do this helps you to relax.

MASSAGE

Not only does gentle massage relieve tension and aid relaxation, but it can also alleviate the minor discomforts of pregnancy such as headaches and backache.

If you can, have a regular massage during pregnancy by a trained massage therapist. You could also ask your husband to give you a massage, which is a good way of staying close to each other physically. Basic massage techniques are not difficult to learn: you (or he) should buy an instruction book or tape and practice the gentler strokes until he is confident.

For a quick stress beater, try massaging your own shoulders.

1 Start with your upper arm and gently knead and squeeze your muscle to loosen any "knots." Start with light pressure and gradually build up until you can feel tension leaving the muscles.

2 Use smooth circular movements as you work up your arm to your shoulder. Use your whole hand to cup your shoulder, and gently squeeze the muscles of your upper back and shoulder.

3 Finally, with your fingertips gently stroke the muscles at the side of your neck into your hairline.

Repeat as many times as necessary to eliminate all tension in one shoulder, then repeat on the other shoulder.

3

INSTANT STRESS BEATERS

When it all gets too much, or you are particularly busy but feel you do not have enough time to stop and relax properly, reduce tension in one of these ways.

■ 5–10 minute break: Sit in a comfortable chair or lie on the floor (but do not lie flat on your back during the late stages of pregnancy). Close your eyes and take a deep and slow breath in through your nose and out through your mouth. Systematically tense or stretch all parts of your body, then let go. Try to empty your mind of all thoughts.

■ 2-minute break: Sit on a chair, and breathing slowly and deeply let yourself go limp and floppy like a rag doll.

■ When you have no time: Take a few deep breaths, tense your shoulders up to your ears, hold for a second or two, relax them, then roll them back and forth a few times. Close your eyes and screw up your face by frowning hard. Hold for a few seconds. Slowly relax your face feature by feature.

RELAXATION

However much you are longing to be a parent, pregnancy can be stressful. Not only do you have to cope with the physical and emotional demands on your body of supporting a new life, but you may have other worries, such as pressure at work or financial concerns which can cause stress. Learning to relax or "switch off" is one of the most effective ways of reducing stress. Below are several stress-reducing exercises and strategies you can practice. But always remember, if you are seriously worried or stressed about anything, talking to a professional counselor may also help.

SIMPLE SWITCHING OFF STRATEGIES

■ Talk to a friend or your spouse; you may be worrying unneccessarily about a problem to which they can see an easy solution.

■ Go for a walk or swim; exercise causes your body to produce endorphins, the so-called "happy" hormones.

■ Go to the movies or the theater, or get engrossed in a good book.

■ Listen to some music or watch an absorbing television program or video.

■ Soak in a warm bubble bath; a warm bath before bed raises the body temperature and may help you to sleep, which is particularly useful if you are lying awake at night worrying.

■ Have a warm shower and visualize the stress running out of you.

■ Do a relaxation exercise (see right).

■ Go for a massage, ask your spouse to give you a massage, or try self massage (see p.59).

■ Buy an audio or video tape teaching relaxation techniques.

■ Don't fill up on "junk" or sugary food in place of a well-balanced diet. This may give you a temporary lift, but can leave you deficient in nutrients and can add to your stress.

■ Resist the temptation to turn to a cigarette or to alcohol to relieve your stress.

BREATHING AND RELAXATION

The natural reaction to tension or anxiety is to alter our normal breathing pattern, to take rapid, shallow, and irregular breaths into the upper part of the chest. This is known as hyperventilation, and it can cause dizziness and aggravate feelings of anxiety. If it happens in labor, it can also increase any feelings of panic or of being out of control which, in turn, may make it more difficult to cope with contractions in labor and may make labor more painful. Smooth, easy breathing can, on the other hand, help release tension and bring on a state of relaxation. Breathing techniques form an integral part of most prenatal classes.

PRACTICING RELAXATION

1 Wear loose comfortable clothing, choose a warm quiet room, and unplug the phone. Sit comfortably or lie down on a carpet or blanket with your head and neck supported, your legs bent and feet apart (Do not lie flat on your back to relax during the late stages of pregnancy as the baby may press against one of the major blood vessels, restricting blood flow across the placenta and making you feel faint or dizzy.)

2 Unclench your hands so that your fingers curl naturally. Drop your shoulders and relax your jaw. Close your eyes and try to empty your mind of thoughts or visualize a peaceful place. Starting with your toes, tense and relax every part of your body, until your whole body feels limp and heavy.

3 With your lips closed, take a slow, deep breath in through your nose, filling your lungs with air so that you feel your stomach muscles rise. Breathe out gently through your lips in a blowing, sighing motion. Continue until you feel completely relaxed. Try not to let any thoughts arise.

3

4 Consciously concentrate on the rhythm of your breathing, feeling the air flowing into and out of your lungs. Check every so often that your whole body is still relaxed, and if not, tense and relax any areas that are not. When you feel ready to get up, support yourself on your hands and your left knee.

5 Place your left foot flat on the floor and push up with your hands. This is also an ideal way to end a more formal exercise session, or to restore flagging energy levels, perhaps after a day at work, but it takes practice to be able to switch off completely.

REMINDERS

Being under pressure while you are pregnant is bad for you and your baby. Start now to learn strategies to cope when you are feeling stressed. Moderate, regular exercise will make it easier to deal with minor discomforts, help you to sleep, and increase the healthy glow of pregnancy that most women experience, usually in the second trimester.

- Use simple switching-off strategies.
- Don't lie flat on your back after the fourth or fifth month of pregnancy.
- Learn breathing and relaxation exercises.
- Check with your doctor before doing exercise if you have been ill, have had a miscarriage, or have a complicated pregnancy.
- When exercising, be aware of your breathing and never hold your breath.
- Always follow the exercise guidelines, listen to what your body is telling you, and don't push yourself.
- Exercise should be enjoyable, not a chore. Even simple and moderate exercise, such as half an hour's brisk walking a day, is beneficial.
- Make sure that a trained instructor takes your exercise or relaxation class and always inform the instructor that you are pregnant so that he or she can modify the program for your needs, if necessary.
- The recommended duration of aerobic exercise is less than 45 minutes, with strenuous exercise not more than 15 minutes. Do not take up new strenuous exercise during pregnancy.
- Stop exercising and consult your doctor if you experience any of the following symptoms:

  Vaginal bleeding
  A leak or gush of amniotic fluid
  Pain of any kind
  Contractions or abdominal pain
  Nausea, dizziness, or faintness
  Shortness of breath
  Palpitations or very rapid heartbeat
  Any swelling or numbness
  Pain in the legs or difficulty in walking
  Persistent headaches
  Visual disturbances
  Decreased fetal movements
  Excessive tiredness

Prenatal Care, Labor, and Birth

PRENATAL CARE, LABOR, AND BIRTH

While you are pregnant, you will probably receive more medical care and attention than at any other stage of your life. You will be asked to attend regular prenatal checks to chart your baby's growth and development. Several routine procedures will be carried out to confirm that all is well with you, too. If there are complications with your pregnancy or if it falls into the high-risk category, you may be offered more specific tests and be seen more frequently by health-care professionals. If you are not sure what a test is for or whether it is necessary, discuss it further with your doctor.

Your prenatal care, however, is also about preparation for labor and birth. Most births are routine, but sometimes intervention is necessary. A part of good care is to prepare you to cope with every eventuality in the labor room and to understand what is happening at each stage. Some parents-to-be and their caregivers formalize all these discussions by making a birth plan.

4

CHECKS FOR YOU

During pregnancy your health will be monitored regularly. Ideally, you will probably be asked to attend monthly check-ups until 28 to 32 weeks, then every two weeks until 36 weeks, then weekly until delivery. A number of tests may be carried out to make sure that everything is all right. Some of these are routine, others may be special tests offered if problems occur or you are considered to be at risk, for example, if you are over 35, or if you have a family history of medical conditions that could affect your pregnancy (see pp. 68–69). If there is anything that you don't understand, don't be afraid to ask your doctor to explain. Use the Personal File (pp.104–105) to jot down questions and to keep your own pregnancy record.

BLOOD TESTS

BLOOD GROUP AND RH (RHESUS) FACTOR
A blood sample will be taken to test for your blood group in case a transfusion is needed later and for your Rh or Rhesus factor. If you are Rh negative, and your baby is Rh positive, you will be given medication so that your blood will not produce antibodies that fight your baby's blood.

RUBELLA IMMUNITY
Your doctor will check if you are immune to rubella (German measles). Not being immune can be dangerous in the first three months of pregnancy (see p. 8).

HEMOGLOBIN LEVELS
Your blood will be checked for levels of hemoglobin (red blood cells) to check whether you are anemic. If levels are very low, iron may be prescribed.

DISEASES AND DISORDERS
Hepatitis B, HIV virus, and syphilis can be indicated by a blood test. Genetic disorders such as sickle cell anemia and thalassemia (see p. 9) will be tested for if you are at risk of being a carrier.

GLUCOSE TOLERANCE
Some doctors ask their patients to take a high glucose drink at approximately 28 weeks (earlier if there is a family history or other risk factor) to test for "gestational" diabetes. If a blood sample reveals an abnormally high level of glucose, you may be treated as diabetic while you are pregnant.

4

YOUR FIRST PRENATAL VISIT

You will probably have your first and longest prenatal check between 6 and 12 weeks of pregnancy when your doctor will take down a detailed family history.

In addition to the tests carried out at every visit, you will be given a physical examination and an internal examination.

PHYSICAL EXAMINATION

Your doctor will check your heart, lungs, and breasts, and make sure your general health is good. Your height will also be checked – if you are small, you may have a small pelvis which may make a vaginal delivery more difficult and the possibility of a cesarean birth may be discussed.

INTERNAL EXAMINATION

Your doctor may do this to confirm your pregnancy and the size of your uterus or you may be offered an early ultrasound scan (see pp. 68–69). A Pap smear may also be carried out to check for any cell abnormalities, and a swab test may be done to check for sexually transmitted diseases (STD) such as Chlamydia or Gonorrhea. Other tests include Yeast, Trichomonas and Bacterial Vaginosis.

AT EVERY VISIT

BLOOD PRESSURE

This will be monitored to check that it is normal. If it rises significantly, it can be a sign of preeclampsia (very high blood pressure). You will be advised to rest, and your doctor will monitor you closely.

URINE

This will be tested for sugar and protein. Sugar may indicate diabetes (many women develop diabetes in pregnancy; it disappears after the birth.) Traces of protein may mean you have an infection, or it can be a sign of preeclampsia. Urinalysis and a urine culture may also be checked.

4

WEIGHT

This will be monitored at every visit. A gain of between 22–35 pounds (10–16.5kg) is normal, but a sudden large weight gain can indicate preeclampsia or diabetes.

PALPATION

Your abdomen will be felt so that the size and position of your baby can be checked, and the fetal heartbeat is checked as soon as it is audible. Your baby's heartbeat can be heard at 10–11 weeks with a hand-held ultrasound or at 20 weeks with a fetoscope (a special stethoscope).

HOW BABIES DEVELOP

Doctors date pregnancy from your last menstrual period, so that about two weeks after conception, you are termed "four weeks pregnant." The average pregnancy lasts about 40 weeks, although a baby born after 37 weeks is considered "term." Even in the womb babies develop at different rates, but if your baby seems to have stopped growing, your doctor will check for a reason. Most first-time mothers do not recognize their babies' earliest movements (second-time mothers are more sure). If you do not feel your baby move by about week 21, or your baby has started to move and then seems to stop, contact your doctor for further advice. The chances are that a quiet spell means that your baby is asleep, but it always worth checking if you are concerned.

6 weeks

4-6 weeks

Your baby will have buried itself into the lining of your uterus by the fourth week of pregnancy and is the size of a pinhead. At 6 weeks, the baby is about ¼ inch (6mm) long, and the head, body, and "limb buds" have formed.

8 weeks

8–10 weeks

Your baby's heart is now beating 140 to 150 times a minute and can be picked up on ultrasound. She has grown to ½ –1 inch (13–25mm) long, and her major organs (heart, lungs, liver, and kidneys) are almost formed. Her eyes, ears, fingers, and toes are in their correct position and nearly formed.

9 weeks

4

11–12 weeks

Your baby's most vulnerable stage is almost over, since most of her major organs, including the sex organs, are formed. But it is still impossible to tell the baby's gender on an ultrasound scan. Her head is becoming more rounded, and her kidneys have started to function. She is now about 3 inches (75mm) long.

16 weeks

15–16 weeks

By 16 weeks your baby has developed fingers and toes, can make facial expressions, suck her fingers, and drink in some of the amniotic fluid and pass it out through the bladder. A fine hair called lanugo covers the whole body. She now weighs about 4 ounces (125g). You may even feel the first "butterfly" type movements from your baby. The time a women first becomes aware of her baby's movements is often called "quickening."

18–20 weeks

At around this time, most mothers can definitely feel their baby kicking or moving. You may even be able to see these movements under your skin. She has hair on her head, and her eyebrows and eyelashes have developed. The skin is covered with a white greasy substance called vernix. This protects your baby from the amniotic fluid. Ask your doctor or midwife to check if you have not felt your baby move by 21 weeks.

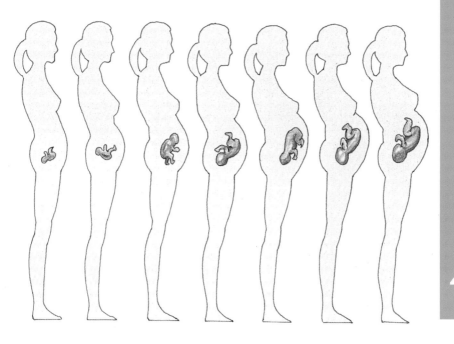

24 weeks

Your baby's skin has started to thicken. She can hear more clearly, and loud sudden noises may make her jump. Her eyes are open, and she has periods of waking and sleeping. Babies born after 24 weeks have a chance of surviving with intensive care. She now weighs about 1¼ pounds (600g) and is about 14 inches (36cm) long.

32 weeks

Her lungs are now mature enough for her to breathe unaided and if born, she has a very good chance of surviving. She weighs about 3 pounds (1,300g) and is about 16 inches (40cm) long.

36–40 weeks

All organs are now fully formed and working normally. At any time from 36 weeks, her head may "engage," or move down into the pelvis. She is now ready to be born.

TESTS FOR YOUR BABY

In addition to the routine tests and check-ups discussed on pages 64–65, some special screening tests may also be carried out to identify a wide range of fetal abnormalities. Not all these tests are available in every hospital and some may be offered only if your baby is thought to be at a high risk from a particular condition. Although most of the tests are perfectly safe, some do carry a small risk of a miscarriage, so you will need to consider this, and the possible implications of the results of the tests, before you agree to a test.

Tests can be divided into screening tests which will indicate the risk to you of having a baby with an abnormality, and diagnostic tests which will tell you whether or not your baby is affected by an abnormality. Most women who have a screening test go on to have normal babies.

ULTRASOUND

An ultrasound scan involves placing a probe over your abdomen. (In early pregnancy, the probe may be placed in the vagina). Sound waves sent to the uterus are reflected back, allowing a moving picture of the fetus to be shown on the screen. Scans measure the size of the fetus and identify some physical signs of abnormalities. (It may also be possible to see the genitals, thereby determining the baby's sex; if you don't want to know, say so.) A scan is usually carried out routinely around 18–20 weeks, but may be done earlier to diagnose pregnancy.

Most parents-to-be find their ultrasound scans one of the most thrilling parts of pregnancy as they see their baby moving around in the womb. In some cases you may be offered a photograph of the image; in others a video may be available. If you want one, you may have to ask for it.

4

SELECTIVE TESTS

Alphafetoprotein (AFP)

Here the levels of Alphafetoprotein (AFP), a substance produced by the fetus, are measured in the mother's bloodstream, normally between 15–18 weeks of pregnancy. Higher levels than expected could indicate the pregnancy is more advanced than was thought, may be caused by twins, or may occur if the baby has a neural tube defect, such as spina bifida. Lower levels than expected could indicate the pregnancy is less advanced than believed or Down's syndrome. Follow-up tests will be carried out if necessary.

■ You may be offered further special tests (if available) if your AFP levels seem too high or low, if you are over the age of 35, or if there are other risk factors in your pregnancy. Before having any further diagnostic tests, the implications of them should be explained, and you should receive counseling from your doctor. You are entitled to refuse any tests offered. Current diagnostic tests include:

Chorionic Villus Sampling

■ Involves removing a small sample of cells from the placenta. Carries a higher risk of miscarriage than amniocentesis.

■ This test is usually carried out to detect some serious fetal disorders, such as cystic fibrosis, Down's Syndrome, Tay-Sach's, and sickle cell anemia; but not for spina bifida.

Amniocentesis

■ A sample of amniotic fluid (which has the same genetic makeup as the baby) is withdrawn through the abdomen with a fine needle. Carries a slight risk of miscarriage.

■ The procedure is performed during the 14–18th week of pregnancy. It may be offered when the woman is over 35, or when the family history suggests there may be a risk of fetal abnormalities, chromosomal abnormalities, or genetic disorders.

Triple test

■ This blood test is an extension of the AFP test and is more accurate.

■ There is also a new quadruple test which may be offered in some places, to detect Down's syndrome.

■ The triple test is ideally carried out at 15–19 weeks to detect the risk of Down's and other chromosomal abnormalities.

Cordocentesis (umbilical vein sampling)

■ This examines the blood of the fetus from the umbilical cord. The risk of miscarriage is between 1 and 4 per 100, depending on the unit.

■ Cordocentisis can be carried out from the 18th week of pregnancy to test for infections in the fetus, such as rubella or toxoplasmosis, or if an amniocentesis result is unclear. It can also be used to check for metabolic disorders.

4

MAKING A BIRTH PLAN

There are several ways to approach labor and delivery. A birth plan is a written list of your ideal preferences and priorities, such as who you want your birth companion to be. It is best completed a month to six weeks before your estimated delivery date as this gives you a chance to attend prenatal classes and discuss various issues with your doctor. It is also early enough to negotiate any changes you would like to your caregiver's normal practice. Make sure your birth plan is easy to read and follow (some doctors provide special forms), and date and sign it. One copy of the plan should be clipped to your notes and another kept by you. Be prepared to be flexible if your needs change or if you or your baby's health could be compromised by sticking to your plan. Your spouse or birth companion should be aware of your wishes on your birth plan and help make sure they are carried out. Different things are important to different people, so think through your priorities carefully.

If your husband is not going to be present at the birth, it is best to choose someone who you can rely on, is calm in a crisis, will give you good emotional support, and will not be squeamish at the birth.

4

BIRTH COMPANION

■ Do you wish to have a birth companion, such as your husband, or a friend or relative, with you? If so, can you bring the companion of your choice?

■ Can he or she stay with you throughout labor and delivery, including a cesarean section, if necessary?

■ Is more than one companion allowed?

Example heading:
Birth companion

I would like my sister with me during birth, as well as my husband

DURING LABOR

■ Do you want to walk around freely during labor or would you prefer to be monitored electronically?

■ What kind of pain relief do you want, if any? If you do not want any pain relief, be sure to write this on your plan.

■ Are epidurals available?

■ Can you bring in a complementary medical practitioner, such as an acupuncturist?

Example heading:
Pain relief

I would like to use a TENS machine and have an epidural if necessary

INDUCTION

- What are your views on induction (starting labor artificially)?
- Ask what are the usual circumstances for this?
- What methods are usually used?
- Can you opt out if you prefer to manage without help?

Example heading:
Acceleration

I do not want my membranes artificially ruptured

SPECIAL EQUIPMENT

- If you would like to have music or aromatherapy essences in the birthing room, can you bring these?
- Will there be a mirror available so I can watch the baby being born?

Example heading:
Music

I find music relaxing and wish to bring my own tapes

DURING THE BIRTH

- Do you mind having an episiotomy if necessary, or would you prefer to tear naturally?
- Do you want your baby delivered straight onto your stomach, or washed first?

Example heading:
Episiotomy

I would prefer an episiotomy to tearing

AFTER THE BIRTH

- If you plan to breastfeed, will the baby be put straight to your breast?
- How soon do you wish to go home if you have the choice?

Example heading:
Discharge

I wish to spend only one night in the hospital if all is well

4

CESAREAN SECTION

- Can I have a choice of a general anesthetic or an epidural?
- Can my birth companion or husband stay during the operation if he wishes to?
- If my baby is well enough, can I hold her immediately after birth, or can my birth companion hold her while I recover?

Example heading:
Cesarean section

If I need a cesarean I would prefer an epidural and would like my birth companion to stay

SIGNS OF LABOR

Only five percent of babies are born on the expected date of delivery (EDD). Most women go into labor within two weeks of this date, but it is a good idea to have your hospital bags packed from 36 weeks (see pp.106-107). Although as many babies are born after 40 weeks as before, you may find yourself very tired of waiting once your EDD has come and gone. Your doctor will continue to monitor your baby's health and, if there are no signs that labor is about to start by around 42 weeks, will probably suggest that labor is induced (started artificially).

LIGHTENING AND ENGAGEMENT

Some time during the last four weeks before birth, your baby's head will probably descend into the pelvic cavity ready for delivery. The head is then said to be "engaged." You may notice when this has happened because you will feel less pressure on your chest and upper abdomen and be able to breathe more freely again. This is known as "lightening." In second or subsequent pregnancies, the head may not engage until shortly before labor starts, or even after the membranes have ruptured.

You will feel less pressure on your diaphragm.

About 5 percent of babies do not move into this position and are born with their feet or buttocks first (in a breech position). Some breech babies are delievered vaginally; others by cesarean section.

The head is engaged, well down in the pelvic cavity.

CONTRACTIONS

Some time after the 20th week of pregnancy, you will experience painless tightenings of the uterus. These are known as Braxton Hicks contractions and are thought to help prepare the uterus for labor. They may become stronger and painful near your date of delivery, and may be mistaken for labor pains. True labor contractions, however, increase in intensity and frequency.

You will feel the contractions of early labor as a mild backache or as something like period pains or an aching feeling. You may also be nauseated, actually vomit, or have diarrhea.

WHAT TO DO

Time your contractions. Once they start coming every 5—10 minutes, lasting 30 seconds or longer, call your doctor. At first, contractions may be irregular, but will gradually become stronger and more frequent.

4

START OF LABOR

In additon to contractions, there are two easy-to-recognize signs that mark the start of labor. These occur in any order, and may succeed each other quickly, or there may be a few days between them.

■ The "show."

The plug of mucus that has helped to seal the entrance to the uterus during pregnancy comes away. Known as the "show," it is a sticky pinkish discharge, but there should not be a lot of blood.

WHAT TO DO

If you are losing blood, call your doctor immediately. Otherwise, wait for contractions to start or your water to break.

■ The water breaking (rupture of membranes).

The bag of amniotic fluid that surrounded your baby during pregnancy breaks, and the water comes out in a gush or a trickle, depending on the size of the tear and the position of the baby's head.

WHAT TO DO

If this happens, phone the hospital, or your doctor. You will probably be advised to go to the hospital at once, even if there are no contractions, as your baby is no longer protected against infection.

WHEN SHOULD I GO TO THE HOSPITAL?

When to go into the hospital depends on what you have been advised by your doctor, how far you live from the hospital, and how anxious you are. But a first labor may take quite a long time, and you will probably feel more relaxed if you stay at home for the first few hours. In early labor, try to keep moving around and have something light to eat and drink to keep your strength up. Practice your relaxation techniques, time your contractions every so often, and – if your membranes have not ruptured – have a warm bath or shower.

4

Warning!

If any of the signs of labor listed above occur before you are 36 weeks pregnant, call your doctor immediately.
If labor is very premature, treatment may be given to try to stop it.

THE FIRST STAGE

There are three stages of labor which, for the birth of a first baby, lasts on average 12 to 14 hours. The first stage is the longest and from the start of established labor usually lasts 6 to 10 hours. During this time, contractions become progressively stronger and gradually shorten the muscles of the cervix, pulling it upward (called effacement and measured in percentages) and open (called dilatation and measured in centimeters) to allow the baby to descend the birth canal.

AT THE HOSPITAL

Once you arrive at the hospital, your doctor or midwife will:
- Ask you about the start of your labor
- Check your pulse, temperature, blood pressure, and urine
- Examine your cervix to check how far it has dilated.

MONITORING YOUR BABY'S HEART RATE

Throughout labor your baby's heart rate will be monitored. It is usual for a baby's heart rate to dip as your contraction reaches its peak intensity, then to pick up as the contraction subsides. But any change from this pattern could indicate that your baby is not coping well with labor (this is termed "in distress"). If the baby is distressed, action may be needed to speed delivery. Monitoring may be done by :

INTERMITTENT AUSCULTATION(IA)

Here a special stethoscope called a "Pinard" or a handheld ultrasound machine called a "Doppler" is used every 15–30 minutes throughout labor and more often during the second stage. With this method you can move about freely.

ELECTRONIC FETAL MONITORING (EFM)

The fetal heart rate is measured for 10–30 minutes every two to four hours or continuously throughout labor by a monitor strapped by a belt to your abdomen, or an electrode attached to your baby's scalp. You cannot easily move around with this method, unless your hospital uses a remote control system called telemetry. A TENS machine for pain relief (see pp. 76–77) may prevent an EFM from working properly.

COPING DURING LABOR

There are no hard and fast rules about what position to adopt during labor, the main thing is that you are as relaxed and comfortable as possible. You may wish to squat, sit, kneel, lie down, or use a mixture of positions. But unless you have to stay in bed for medical reasons, being upright – walking around, standing, sitting, squatting, or kneeling – is less painful and may shorten labor.

4

SITTING

There is no way of knowing how long labor will last, so conserving your strength makes sense. Sit between contractions to rest. Lean forward to keep up pressure on the cervix, and relieve pressure on your lower back. If you need extra support during a contraction, lean against the back of a chair. Place a pillow on the back to rest your head between contractions.

KNEELING

Kneeling as you lean forward on your arms takes pressure off the cervix. This may slow labor, but can be useful when contractions start to come close together. It also relieves pressure on your back, which can be painful.

STANDING

Early in labor standing and walking around between contractions keeps the pressure on your cervix, helping the contractions to dilate it. Lean against a wall or your birth partner for support during a contraction. Your partner can also massage your back in this position.

4

PAIN RELIEF IN LABOR

There are different forms of pain relief available should you need it. Knowing what is available will help you to make the best choice for you and your baby.

SELF HELP

■ Practice the breathing and relaxation techniques you learned in your prenatal class.

■ Get plenty of rest at the end of your pregnancy, and in the early stages of labor rest as much as you can. You will find it harder to cope with pain if you are physically or emotionally exhausted.

■ Don't hold your breath during a contraction, but breathe through the pain by keeping your shoulders and jaw loose, and breathing out. Try not to tense as a contraction peaks – tension leads to pain.

■ Think positively when having a contraction – remind yourself that each one is bringing the birth of your baby nearer.

■ Listen to your body and adopt the position most comfortable for you.

■ If your back aches, try applying a hot-water bottle or heating pad.

■ Don't be embarrassed by making noises such as grunting to help you cope.

■ Choose a practical, but sympathetic birthing partner. Most women choose their husbands (and most men want to be there for the birth of their child), but discuss with him ahead of time how he will handle the fact that you are in pain. If you think he is not going to offer the help you need, talk about it together before you go into labor.

■ Ask your birthing partner to give you a massage.

■ Create a relaxed atmosphere by playing music, or ask for the lights to be dimmed.

DRUGFREE PAIN RELIEF

If you don't want to use drugs during labor, you still have choices for pain relief.

TENS

Some hospitals may have a TENS (Transcutaneous Electrical Nerve Stimulation) machine. This involves the use of electrodes attached to the lower back. These stimulate nerve endings in the skin to trigger the release of the body's own pain-relieving substances. They also prevent pain signals from traveling to the brain. For some women, TENS can be very effective, and it allows you to be in control, but it needs to be started early in labor. If your hospital does not have a TENS machine, you may be able to rent one. (Do this in advance to practice with it.)

BREATHING AND RELAXATION

Many prenatal approaches (see p. 19) are based on breathing and relaxation exercises. If you want to follow the approach of Fernand Lamaze or Robert Bradley, it is important for you and your husband to start taking classes together early in pregnancy.

DRUGS FOR PAIN RELIEF

Some women prefer not to have drugs during labor and delivery, others like to see how their labor progresses before they take a final decision. Keep in mind that every woman is different, and what one can cope with, another cannot. In addition, some studies have shown that women who use drugs wisely in labor, are less likely to suffer from "failure to progress" and therefore less likely to need a cesarean.

If you are concerned about your ability to handle pain, talk in advance with your doctor and have all your options explained clearly. Then, when you go into labor, you will be able to make wise decisions about what help you need.

EPIDURAL

This is an anesthetic injected between two spinal vertebrae in the lower back (see below), which numbs the nerves. It removes pain and can be used for an elective cesarean. In some women, it lowers the blood pressure (but you can be given drugs to prevent this), may affect their legs and bladder for a while, and may cause headaches afterward. Some babies born after an epidural are drowsy, but the breathing problems associated with painkillers such as Demerol do not occur after an epidural.

DEMEROL/STADOL/NUBAIN

This drug is given by injection and relieves pain. It may be combined with a tranquilizer for a calming effect, or with other drugs to relieve nausea (which many women experience after a shot). If given too near the second stage, it may make it harder for you to push effectively, and can make your baby sleepy or depress her breathing. Rarely, a baby may need oxygen for a few hours after the birth. Your dose will be monitored very carefully to minimize these problems.

4

Epidural

One of the major criticisms of epidurals was that they affected a woman's ability to push during the second stage of labor, making a forceps delivery more likely. However, doses can now be controlled so precisely and are administered early, with the result that most women have enough feeling back by the second stage that they can actively participate in the delivery.

Spine

Site of epidural injection

Vertebrae

THE SECOND STAGE

The second stage begins when your cervix is fully dilated (at 4in/10cm) and ends when your baby is born. It lasts an average of 60 minutes with the first labor, but may take as little as 10 minutes, or as much as two hours. Most doctors intervene if it goes on for longer than two hours (or three hours if you have an epidural).

TRANSITION

This is the stage between the late part of the first stage and the beginning of the second, and is the most exhausting and challenging period of labor. It may be very brief or last for an hour or more. Your cervix is almost fully dilated, and contractions are very strong, long, and frequent.

■ During this time you may feel hot and sweaty or cold and shivery, or alternate between the two. Your legs may feel cold and tremble, and you may feel nauseated or even vomit. Tell your birth partner what you need – socks, cracked ice to suck, a warm blanket, a cool sponge.

■ You are likely to feel a powerful urge to push or bear down. Unless you have been told to push by your doctor or midwife, it is important not to. Pushing before the cervix is fully dilated can cause it to become swollen, making it difficult for the baby to pass through the opening. It may also tear the cervix.

■ To prevent yourself from bearing down, kneel with your buttocks in the air. This takes the pressure of the baby's head off your cervix, which slightly reduces the urge to push. It also helps you to conserve your energy for the second stage.

4

WHAT YOUR BIRTH COMPANION CAN DO

■ Encourage you and remind you to take one contraction at a time.

■ Help you to focus on how far you have come, and how many contractions are behind you.

■ Check your needs and talk or touch only if this helps; mood swings are normal, especially during transition, and your needs will change from moment to moment.

■ Mop your brow with a cool damp cloth, if this helps.

■ Once you are given the okay to push, help your efforts to concentrate. Pushing assists a contraction, pushing between them wastes your efforts.

■ Be there for you: you are likely to push him away at least once; he should take it all with good grace.

POSITIONS FOR THE SECOND STAGE

Once your cervix is fully dilated, you can adopt the position you find most comfortable and effective for pushing and delivery. It is much easier if you can adopt an upright position because gravity makes it easier for your baby to pass down the birth canal.

KNEELING

Kneeling is almost as good for widening the pelvis. You can hang onto your partner's neck, or your partner and the nurse can support you under your arms.

SUPPORTED SQUAT

Squatting is one of the best ways to widen the pelvis and allow gravity to push your baby out. Your partner can kneel behind you to support you under the arms, or sit behind you. You could also try a semisquat, standing with your knees bent, while your partner supports you.

4

STANDARD DELIVERY POSITION

This is one of the most common delivery positions. You sit in a semi-upright position with your back supported, either on pillows or with your partner sitting behind you. Your knees should be drawn up with your legs wide apart and your hands against the back of your thighs. In this position you can hold a mirror to your vagina to see the baby's head as it emerges.

BIRTH

The nine months of waiting are now almost over, and you will soon meet your baby. If you are having a "normal delivery," your baby will be born head first without any extra help. Sometimes, however, a cesarean or other type of delivery may become necessary.

PUSHING DURING THE SECOND STAGE

To push your baby out, breathe deeply while your contraction is building up, then as it reaches a peak, push for about five seconds, or until you want to take a breath (holding your breath unnecessarily can exhaust you and may reduce the oxygen content in your baby's blood.) If the contraction is still peaking, take a few deep breaths and push again. You will probably have the urge to push three to five times in each contraction. As you push, your baby's head will become visible at each contraction, and then slip back a little in between. You may be given an episiotomy – a small cut into the perineum, the skin between the vagina and rectum, to prevent it tearing at the time the baby is crowning (see below). If you do not want an episiotomy, then you can state this on your birth plan.

THE MOMENT OF BIRTH

When your baby is about to be born, her head will appear at the vaginal opening and no longer slip back – this is known as "crowning" (the skin of your perineum "crowns" her head). You may then be asked not to push but to pant instead, as your baby's head is gently guided out. At this stage you may wish to use a mirror to see the birth, or your partner may wish to videotape it. Suction may be applied to your baby's mouth and nose to remove excess mucus. Another push may be needed for the shoulders and rest of the body to glide out. If your baby is not breathing, further suction or oxygen may be required. But if everything is normal, your baby may be put on your stomach while the umbilical cord is being cut, or you may be able to hold your baby immediately.

4

The head crowns and is clearly visible to your caregivers.

With one more contraction the head emerges.

ASSISTED DELIVERY

If your second stage is particularly difficult or prolonged, the doctor may remove the baby with the help of forceps or a vacuum extractor. With forceps, after a local anesthetic, two metal blades that look like tongs are inserted into the vagina, one at a time. These cradle the head, and the baby is drawn from the birth canal. With a vacuum extractor, a plastic or metal cup is attached to the head, and traction is applied to assist delivery. An episiotomy may be needed if either method is used, but their use may avoid the need for a cesarean section.

CESAREAN BIRTH

About one in four babies are born by cesarean section. Sometimes a cesarean can be planned in advance if your doctor considers it necessary (an elective cesarean), or it may become necessary as labor proceeds. The reasons for a cesarean include:

■ Your baby needs delivering quickly if, for example, there is fetal distress, you have had a hemorrhage, or if you have a medical condition such as preeclampsia or diabetes.

■ Your baby is awkwardly positioned, such as a breech or transverse (shoulder first) position.

■ Your baby is large and her head is stuck in the pelvis, which is too narrow.

■ Your labor is not progressing for some reason.

■ The placenta is lying across the cervix.

■ You are having more than one baby.

■ You have active genital herpes which could infect the baby during a vaginal birth.

THE PROCEDURE
Before the operation your pubic hair will be shaved, a catheter inserted in your bladder, and an intravenous infusion started in case you need medication during the delivery. You may be given a choice of a general anesthetic (you will be unconscious) or an epidural or spinal block (you will be awake during the delivery but the lower part of your body will be numb). In an emergency, a general anesthetic may be needed for speed.

An incision will be made in your lower abdomen and uterus, and your baby will be removed manually or with forceps. Your baby will be checked and might be given to you or your husband to hold while you are stitched.

Site of cesarean incision

4

THE THIRD STAGE

The third stage of labor is the shortest. It consists of expelling the placenta or afterbirth from the lining of your uterus once your baby has been born, and usually lasts from around five minutes to about half an hour. During this time you will continue to have contractions, although they will be less intense and, in the excitement of getting to know your baby, you may not feel them.

DELIVERY OF THE PLACENTA

As your baby is being born, you will probably be given a routine injection – usually in the thigh – of a hormone preparation called oxytocin. You may not feel this being done. (Proponents of natural childbirth argue against the routine use of oxytocin; oxytocin is produced by your body in response to your baby's sucking at your breast. If your baby starts to suck right away synthetic oxytocin may be unnecessary.)

Oxytocin helps the uterus to contract and expel the placenta. Once the placenta has detached itself from the uterus, the doctor or midwife may gently pull on the cord to remove the placenta and ask you to help by pushing or bearing down. After the placenta is removed, it will be examined to make sure that it is intact and that no fragments are left inside, which can cause unnecessary bleeding and infection.

Your perineum will then be stitched if you have had a tear or an episiotomy. Try to be patient while this is happening; the doctor or nurse will work as quickly as they can. Your temperature, pulse, blood pressure, uterus, and lochia (vaginal bleeding) will be checked, and you will be made comfortable. Then you will be left with your baby and husband or birth companion to get some rest, and to spend some time together as a family.

4

TECHNICAL TERMS

- Active birth – an approach to childbirth that involves moving around and changing positions throughout labor. Delivery is conducted in an "upright" position after learning stretching exercises.
- Amniotic fluid – the fluid surrounding the fetus in the uterus.
- Amniotic sac – the layer of membranes holding the amniotic fluid that surrounds the fetus in the uterus.
- Apgar score – a system used after birth to assess a baby's well-being.
- Bearing down – pushing movement made during the second stage of labor.
- Breech presentation – the buttocks or feet of the baby are facing downward, instead of the head.
- Contractions – regular tightening of uterine muscles to open the cervix to deliver the baby.
- Crowning – the time when the baby's head appears in the vagina and does not slip back again.
- Dilatation – the opening of the cervix in response to uterine contractions.
- EDD – expected date of delivery.
- Embryo – name for the developing baby up to eight weeks of pregnancy.
- Engaged – when the baby's head has settled into the middle of the pelvis.
- Fetal distress – occurs when there is a shortage of oxygen reaching the fetus.
- Fetus – name for the developing baby after the eighth week of pregnancy.
- Fontanelles – two soft spots on the baby's head where the bones have not yet joined.
- Gestation – the length of time between conception and birth.
- Hemorrhage – heavy bleeding. (Antepartum hemorrhage is bleeding before the baby is born, postpartum hemorrhage is bleeding after the baby is born.)
- Induction – artificial starting of labor.
- Lightening – relief from abdominal pressure that follows the engagement of the baby's head.
- Molding – the shaping of the baby's skull as it passes through the vagina.
- Pelvic floor – the "hammock" of muscles that supports the bladder, lower bowel, and uterus
- Perineum – the area of skin between the vagina and rectum.
- Placenta – the organ that provides oxygen and nutrients for the fetus and carries its waste products to the mother's system.
- Preeclampsia – a potentially dangerous condition characterized by high blood pressure; swelling of the hands, face, and feet; sudden and excessive weight gain; and albumin in the urine.
- Protein – Albumin protein is present in tissues and is checked for in urine tests. If present it can be a sign of preeclampsia (high blood pressure).
- Quickening – first fetal moments felt by the mother.
- Uterus (Womb) – the organ in the body in which the baby develops.

4

REMINDERS

In the excitement of your pregnancy, as you watch your shape change to accommodate your growing baby, some things may slip your mind. This checklist will help you to remember the most important parts of your prenatal care, and serve as a quick reminder of what to do during labor and birth.

■ It is essential to keep your prenatal appointments so that any problems or complications can be detected early.

■ If there is anything that you don't understand about your prenatal care, don't be afraid to ask the doctor to explain.

■ Take your prenatal notes or record with you whenever you see the doctor, or if you go away from home, in case you need emergency medical attention.

■ Some special tests carry a slight risk to the fetus. If special tests indicate that there may be fetal abnormalities, you may have to decide whether you want to continue with your pregnancy. If you are not sure what a test is for, or whether it is necessary, discuss this further with your doctor. You are entitled to refuse any test. If tests do indicate an abnormality, you will normally have time to seek counseling before making a final decision.

■ If you do not feel your baby move by 21 weeks or if your baby has started to move and then seems to stop, contact your doctor immediately for advice.

■ Your birth companion does not have to be your spouse, but could be a friend or relative. If you can think of no one you would like to be at the birth, tell your doctor who can arrange for a nurse to support you.

■ If you have preferences for what you would like to happen in labor and delivery, complete your birth plan 4–6 weeks before your expected date of delivery. Be prepared to be flexible if your needs change or if you or your baby's health could be compromised by sticking to your plan.

■ Only 5 percent of babies are born on the expected date of delivery (EDD). Most women go into labor within two weeks either side of this date. It is a good idea to have your hospital bags packed from 36 weeks.

■ The three signs that can be recognized as the start of labor and which can occur in any order are the show, your waters breaking, and contractions.

■ Contractions that do not increase in frequency or intensity are probably not real labor contractions.

■ If your pregnancy lasts longer than about 42 weeks, or labor is prolonged or delayed, the doctor may decide to start or augment it artificially.

■ Every contraction brings you closer to seeing your baby.

■ Nothing you say or do in the labor room will shock, alarm, or distress the medical staff involved in your care.

4

You and Your Baby

YOU AND YOUR BABY

Congratulations. After nine months of anticipation you are now responsible for a tiny baby 24 hours a day – it is not surprising that many parents feel a bit "shellshocked" for the first few weeks. Don't worry: in no time you will be confidently caring for your baby's needs and enjoying his presence in your lives. In the six weeks after the birth, your body will return to its prepregnancy state. Understanding these changes and looking after yourself is an essential part of your own well-being, so eat well, exercise, and rest. If you are in pain or have any problems, don't suffer in silence. Tell your doctor.

In these weeks your baby will change, too: you may see his first smile in this period, you will both learn how rewarding breastfeeding can be, you will start to interpret his cries, and anticipate his needs. Above all, you will enjoy learning how to be a parent.

5

POSTPARTUM CARE

Unless your baby was born by cesarean section, you will probably stay in the hospital for one to two days. When you go home, you need to be aware of what is normal after birth, and when you should check with your doctor.

YOUR PHYSICAL HEALTH

LOCHIA

■ This is the blood and discharge passed from the uterus following birth. It is heavy and red at first, and clots may be passed for 2–4 days. It gradually becomes pinker and lighter and after 2–3 weeks (but sometimes longer) becomes pale and brown, then ceases.

■ Use sanitary pads rather than tampons, as tampons may introduce infection.

■ Tell your doctor if the discharge smells offensive or you have a bright red blood loss or pass clots after the first 4–5 days.

PERINEAL PAIN AND STITCHES

During delivery, the perineum (the area around the vaginal area) often becomes bruised and swollen. You may also have needed stitches. Usually the pain eases once the wound has healed, normally within 7–10 days, but this may sometimes last longer.

■ Ask your doctor for a local anesthetic spray or oral medication for the pain.

■ Bathe the area several times a day with plain warm water. (Or sit in a plastic bowl or baby's bath.) Pat dry with a soft towel, gauze, or soft toilet paper.

■ To help bruising try a pad of chilled witch hazel.

■ Apply an ice pack (a bag of frozen vegetables wrapped in a clean cloth is fine).

■ Drink plenty of fluids to dilute the urine and stop it from stinging.

■ Take measures to prevent constipation (see p. 37).

■ To promote healing, do pelvic floor exercises (see p. 55).

■ Use soft, thick sanitary pads: the thinner ones are harsher.

AFTERPAINS

As your uterus returns to its normal prepregnancy size, you may feel contractionlike pains for the first few days.

■ Try mild analgesics such as acetimenophen or ibuprofen, and relaxation breathing (see p. 60).

■ Avoid codeine, which can cause constipation.

OTHER POSTPARTUM CONCERNS

■ Your period usually resumes six to twelve weeks after delivery. If you are breastfeeding, it may not return for several months.

■ Sexual intercourse is safe as soon as you are healed, and you and your husband are ready, but you may not feel ready for several months. Try to stay close physically even if you do not want to make love.

■ Although sex may be sore at first, it should not hurt. If it does, ask your doctor to check for any problems. Use a lubricating jelly or different positions.

■ Even if you have not had a period or are breastfeeding, if you have sex, you can still get pregnant. Ask your doctor for contraceptive advice.

CESAREAN SECTION

After a cesarean, it is normal to have abdominal pain and discomfort at first, but you should be offered adequate pain relief and extra help in caring for your baby. To help your general recovery, you will be encouraged to move around as soon as possible, and to do breathing and leg exercises (see pp. 56–57). Your wound will probably be checked at about four weeks.

POSTPARTUM EXERCISES

You're feeling exhausted. Your stitches are hurting. The baby's just stopped crying and you want to rest. The last thing you may feel like doing are postpartum exercises. However, gentle exercises really will help to improve circulation, give you some energy, and help get flabby muscles back into shape, which may boost your morale. Turn to pages 56–57 for a reminder about how to do these.

5

POSTPARTUM CHECK

About four to six weeks after the birth, you should have a postpartum check by your doctor when you can discuss any problems. But if you are worried in any way, make an appointment before then. All women recover from childbirth differently, so don't take what anyone else is feeling as an indicator of your health.

POSTPARTUM EMOTIONS

It is normal to feel a mixture of emotions in the first days and weeks after having a baby. You may feel "out of touch" with your body, exhausted after delivery and with meeting the demands of a new baby, and confused about your feelings for your baby and your husband. During this period, it is important that you are kind to yourself, listen to your body, and give yourself time to recover.

FEELING BLUE?

Most mothers suffer from mood swings or the "baby blues" about three to five days after birth, when they feel weepy, angry, or depressed. This is thought to be due to a sudden fall in hormone levels. If the "blues" don't go away within a week or two, or get worse, talk to your doctor; you may be suffering from postpartum depression.

POSTPARTUM DEPRESSION

This is an extremely distressing condition which is thought to affect at least one woman in ten. Although it usually appears within 2–8 weeks after birth, it can appear up to six months or even a year after the birth. Many women are reluctant to admit to postpartum depression, or they may deny their symptoms. However, effective treatment is available, and if you feel you are suffering from postpartum depression, it is essential that you seek help.

■ Signs and symptoms include:

   crying and anxiety
   panic attacks
   sleeplessness
   aches and pains
   lethargy (all new parents are tired, but the lethargy that may accompany
      postpartum depresssion is different; you may deel unable to make a cup of
      coffee or answer the phone, for example)
   feeling unable to cope, either with the baby or with any other aspect of your
      life
   indifference toward the baby, or frequent concern about the baby
   memory loss
   feelings of unreality
   loss of self esteem
   loss of appetite or excessive appetite
   inability to concentrate
   antagonism toward your husband.

■ Your husband may realize that you are suffering from postpartum depression before you do. If he is concerned about you, take his concerns seriously. The sooner you seek help, the faster you are likely to recover.

■ Treatment includes support, counseling, and perhaps medication.

5

COPING WITH TIREDNESS

Many mothers find the first few weeks of looking after a new baby a shock to the system. Constant feeding and changing, snatched meals and broken nights, plus lots of well-meaning visitors, can leave you feeling exhausted. Things really will get better as you find yourself getting used to your baby, getting into a routine, and regaining your energy. To help you beat tiredness:

■ Get plenty of rest. Unplug the phone if necessary.

■ Limit visitors and make sure they entertain themselves. Put a note on your door if you do not want to be disturbed.

■ Only do essential housework; if you can, pay for some help.

■ Don't be a martyr and feel you have to do everything yourself. Accept any help that is offered, or if necessary, ask for it.

■ Practice relaxation techniques you learned during pregnancy (see pp.58–61).

■ Do something that makes you feel good – have a massage, haircut, or go for a walk or swim by yourself.

■ Don't neglect eating. A good, well-balanced diet is just as important now as it was in pregnancy. Try to avoid "junk foods" and remember, healthy snacks are nourishing and easy to prepare if you haven't yet time or appetite for cooked meals (see p.31 for ideas).

YOU AND YOUR SPOUSE

Adjusting to your new relationship as parents is not always easy. Try to spend a little time together each day to talk about your feelings and have physical contact, even if you do not make love.

WHAT FATHERS CAN DO

■ Get to know your baby. Cuddle, talk, bathe, and change her. Parenthood is a shared experience.

■ Feed the baby if she is bottlefed or support your wife if she is breastfeeding.

■ Take the baby for a walk in the stroller to spend time with her and give your wife a break.

■ Help as much as possible with household chores. If you cook a meal, cook double and freeze half for another day.

■ Make allowances for your wife's changing emotions, but if you think she may be depressed, seek help.

5

YOUR NEW BABY

Seeing a newborn for the first time can be quite a shock. Although it is rarely a disappointment for parents, you may have mentally pictured a smooth-cheeked dream baby as portrayed in advertisements. Instead, you may have a baby who is covered with a white waxy substance, with a wrinkled red face, and perhaps some other strange features that you feel concerned about. Before you start to worry, be reassured that very few babies look perfect at birth, and most irregularities will disappear within a few weeks. Your baby will also be checked at birth to make sure that everything is all right.

FIRST CHECKS

Checks carried out immediately after birth by the doctor or nurse include:

■ Apgar score: this is used to assess breathing, heart rate, reflexes, skin color, and muscle tone, at one minute and five minutes after birth. The baby is given a rating of 0, 1, or 2 for each measure, which are then combined. A very low rating will merit immediate medical intervention, but a low score is not necessarily a cause for alarm. Few normal babies achieve the maximum score of 10, even after five minutes.

■ Weight, head circumference, and length.

■ A check from head to toe, including the mouth to make sure there is no cleft palate, and the hips for any dislocation.

■ Before leaving the hospital, your baby will also be given a physical examination by the doctor, including the heart and lungs, abdomen, hips, and reflexes.

REFLEXES

Your baby is born with several reflex actions that are early protection measures. The strongest of these are rooting and sucking, which help her to feed (see pp. 98–99). If you put your finger in her hand, she will grasp this tightly (grasp reflex). Or if she is scared, she will fling her arms and legs wide (Moro or startle reflex).

Moro, or startle reflex   Grasp reflex

5

Fontanelles

These are the "soft spots" on the top of the head where the scalp bones have not yet joined together. It is normal for them to beat. The back fontanelle closes in about 6–8 weeks, and the larger front fontanelle gradually closes by 18 months.

Eyes

The eyes may be sticky and swollen at first. See p.96 for advice on cleaning.

Skin

Many babies are covered in vernix, a white greasy substance which protects the baby from the amniotic fluid in the womb. This can be washed off or left to absorb. If your baby was overdue, the skin may be dry or flaky.

Genitals

Some boys may have fluid around the testicles, and girls sometimes have a white or blood-stained discharge from the vagina. Both conditions will disappear without treatment.

Cord

The cord stump shrivels and usually falls off in about a week to ten days; your doctor will advise you on keeping it clean. Tell your doctor if there is any bleeding or discharge.

Breasts

Both sexes sometimes have swollen breasts, and there may be a milky discharge. These are due to the effects of your hormones and will disappear without treatment over a few weeks.

Head

A baby's head is large in proportion to the rest of the body. It is common for it to be misshapen, and there may be a soft bump or a cystlike swelling due to pressure of the head on the dilating cervix. These are all temporary and will disappear over a few weeks.

BOWELS

The stools change over a few days from greeny/black meconium to a greenish-brown color, then yellow color. They are often runny in breastfed babies; bottlefed babies usually have larger, firmer stools. The number of stools passed varies. As long as they are soft and a normal color, there is no need to worry if the bowels are not moved every day or if they are moved several times a day.

WEIGHT

It is normal for babies to lose some weight during the first few days. This is usually regained within 10–14 days.

5

BRINGING BABY HOME

Many mothers are discharged from the hospital within 48 hours of giving birth, before having time to learn basic childcare skills. It can be quite frightening to start looking after your baby yourself, so before leaving the hospital, try to learn as much about baby care as you can. A midwife or other caregiver may be available to visit your home to give you further help and advice. If these services are not available to you, check whether your insurance will cover a home consultation with a visiting nurse. Although caring for your baby is a demanding, 24-hour job, it is also infinitely rewarding. And as you get to know each other and you become skilled in handling your baby, your confidence will grow.

THE RIDE HOME

Going home from the hospital, the baby must be securely strapped in an appropriate car seat. It is not safe to carry your baby on your lap. The car seat must comply with government safety standards and be fitted to the manufacturer's instructions. Infants should use a rear-facing seat until they are 12 months old and weigh at least 20 pounds (10kg). **The car seat must be fitted to a rear seat, not to a front seat.**

GETTING ORGANIZED

The basic needs of a new baby are food, sleep, warmth, and loving attention. Babies rarely feed and sleep following a schedule during the first few weeks, and the only way they have to express their needs is by crying. Although you will eventually get into a daily routine, expect the first few weeks to be hectic and haphazard, and decide on your priorities. It will help you enormously if you can sleep or rest when your baby sleeps and eat in between her feedings, rather than trying to fit her into your schedule. The first few weeks do not set a pattern for the rest of her infancy, so don't worry that she will never settle into a routine.

■ Routines should be flexible and realistic, and will change as your baby grows.

■ Don't try to keep to a timetable for feeding your baby, but let her feed on demand. This will help you to get breastfeeding well established. She will eventually get into her own routine.

■ Don't try to keep your young baby awake during the day so that she will sleep at night – she needs to sleep when she wants to. As she gets older, a routine will emerge.

5

FEELINGS FOR YOUR BABY

You may be overjoyed by the birth and already overwhelmed by love for your baby. Or you may feel very protective of this vulnerable new being, without actually feeling love. Some may have had a difficult birth and need a little time to get themselves on an even keel before they can really start to relate to their babies. If you feel detached or don't feel any love for her, don't panic or feel guilty. Although it is important that you and your baby enjoy a warm and loving relationship, many mothers and fathers do not fall in love or "bond" with their baby at first. Like other relationships, some get off to a slower start than others and need time to grow. The word "bonding" implies that love is like a glue, instantly applied and permanent, but relationships simply are not like that. If you are worried about your feelings for your baby, talk to your doctor or midwife.

SIBLING JEALOUSY

If you have a toddler or child, try to prepare him as much as possible for the arrival of the baby. But even if he seems pleased and affectionate toward her, don't be surprised if he is jealous, if he regresses to an earlier stage of behavior, or exhibits behaviors such as being demanding, clinging, or defiant.

■ When he meets the baby, have a present ready "from the baby." It helps if he can come to the hospital to "bring her home."

■ Ask visitors to make a fuss over your toddler before the baby.

■ Give your toddler extra cuddles and reassurance that you love him.

■ Involve him in helping with the baby as much as possible if he wants to, but if he sees it as a chore, rather than a sign of maturity, don't force it.

■ Reinforce his maturity by letting him decide if he wants to go to playgroup, choose what he wants for lunch, or what he would like to wear.

■ Jealousy is normal.

PETS

Don't invest in a pet if you've just had a baby – looking after two newcomers can be difficult. If you already have a pet, follow the guidelines listed below to avoid passing on any infections to your baby:

■ Let a vet check your pet before the baby is born. Make sure your pet has the necessary shots, is dewormed regularly, and is free from fleas.

■ If you have a dog, discourage it from licking your baby's face.

■ If you have a cat, buy a net for your baby's bed and stroller so the cat can't get in.

■ If you know your pet is likely to be jealous of the baby, make sure the two are never left alone together.

5

BASIC BABY CARE

When picking your baby up, whether to change, bathe, or feed her, always hold her firmly and confidently and talk to her softly and gently, making eye contact.

PICKING UP YOUR BABY

Holding and cuddling your baby makes her feel safe and loved, but this may not come naturally at first, and you may feel nervous.

1 Standing facing her, slide one hand under her head and neck and the other beneath her lower back and bottom.

2 Lift her gently and slowly toward your chest. Turn her so that her head is cradled in the crook of your elbow and her body supported along the length of your arm.

3 When you put her down, support her head and bottom. Slide your hand out from under her bottom first, then from beneath her head.

HOLDING YOUR BABY

There are several ways that babies like to be held, but a newborn baby cannot support her head, so always support her neck to stop her head from flopping back. If you need to keep your arms free but want to keep your baby in close contact with you, try using a sling (see p. 109).

1 Cuddle her close against your shoulder with one hand supporting the head and neck, and the other under her bottom. Hold her upright to look over your shoulder.

2 Cradle her lengthwise in your arms, keeping her head supported.

5

PUTTING ON A SHIRT

Most babies dislike having clothes pulled over their head. You may prefer to buy crossover shirts that tie or snap shut at the side.

1 Gather the shirt at the neck with the front facing you. Place the back of the shirt at the top of your baby's head.

2 Gently raise her head and slip the shirt over her face, taking care not to drag it. Pull the shirt down over her neck and shoulders and lower her down.

3 Gather up the sleeve with one hand, stretch the opening wide, and holding your baby's wrist, guide her arm through. Repeat with the other arm. Pull it down behind her back and do up the snaps under her bottom.

CHANGING YOUR BABY'S DIAPER

To help prevent diaper rash, change your baby's diaper as soon as it becomes wet or soiled. You may find that newborn babies need changing 10–12 times a day.

1 Lie your baby on a changing mat or other flat surface (try to have this at waist height so that you do not have to bend). Remove the old diaper. Lift her legs up by the ankles with one hand and use the old diaper to clean off the worst of any soiling. Roll up the old diaper and put it in a plastic bag.

2 Thoroughly clean the whole area, wiping from front to back with moist cotton balls. Wipes are harsh for a newborn but fine after a couple of months.

3 When her bottom is clean and dry, wash and dry your hands and apply a barrier cream to her bottom. Lift her legs up by the ankles with one hand and slide an opened diaper under her with the other hand. Secure the clean diaper.

5

BASIC BABY CARE

L ooking after your baby will quickly become second nature, but remember that your way will always be slightly different from anybody else's. Baby care is about finding out what works for you and your baby.

"SPONGE BATH"

Your newborn baby does not need a bath every day – once every few days is fine. In between you can keep her clean by giving her a sponge bath. This means undressing your baby a little at a time, and only cleaning the parts that need it, such as her face, hands, and bottom. Never try to clean inside her nose or ears; her mucous membranes are self-cleaning. Just wipe away any visible wax or mucus with damp cotton balls. Use only cooled boiled water and cotton balls – soap will dry her skin, and talcum powder may cause breathing problems.

1 Dip a fresh cotton ball into cooled boiled water and wipe one eye from the nose outward. Repeat with a fresh cotton ball for the other eye. Wipe the skin folds in the neck and under the arms. Pat dry with a soft cloth or towel.

5

2 Put her shirt back on, then use warm water to wash her hands. Undo her diaper and clean her bottom. Pay particular attention to the creases at the top of her thighs. If her toes are tightly curled, gently uncurl them to wipe the soles of her feet. Pat dry with a soft cloth or towel. Let her kick without a diaper for a while, then finish dressing her.

BATHING

1 Collect everything you need before you start, including a waterproof apron, baby toiletries, cotton balls and cooled boiled water, sponge or soft washcloth, clean diaper and clothes.

2 Put cold water in the bathtub first, followed by hot, and test the temperature with your elbow. The water should be warm but not hot.

3 Undress your baby and wrap her snugly in a soft towel across your lap. Wipe her eyes with clean cotton balls dipped in cooled boiled water. Clean around her face and mouth.

4 Wash and rinse her hair, holding her head over the bathtub. Pat her head dry. Unwrap your baby, place one arm under her shoulders, and the other under her bottom, and lower her gently into the bathtub.

5 Supporting her neck and shoulders, wash and rinse her with your free hand. Slide your free arm under her bottom and lift her out gently. Wrap her in a towel and pat her dry. Keep your baby covered while you dress her and put on a clean diaper.

> **Warning**
> Never leave a young baby unattended in the bathtub even for a second. A baby can drown in less than an inch of water.

SLEEPING

Babies vary in the amount of time they sleep, but this is often less than parents expect. On average, new babies may be awake for six to eight hours in every 24 and usually sleep in naps of three to five hours.

CRYING

Crying is your baby's way of telling you she needs something. Gradually, you will learn to distinguish between different cries, such as hunger or tiredness. If your child will not stop crying or appears in pain, contact your doctor.

REDUCING THE RISK OF CRIB DEATH

Sudden infant death syndrome (SIDS), also known as crib death, is rare. However, research suggests there are ways in which you may be able to reduce the risk of this happening:

■ Place your baby on the back to sleep, unless advised otherwise.

■ Don't smoke during pregnancy or after the birth, and do not expose your baby to tobacco smoke or smoky atmospheres.

■ Don't let your baby get too hot. Use light layers of bedclothes.

■ Contact your doctor if you think your baby is unwell.

■ Don't let your baby sleep on a secondhand mattress. Don't use a pillow.

■ Don't let your baby's head get covered by bedclothes. Place her feet at the foot of the bed so that she cannot wriggle down.

5

FEEDING YOUR BABY

How you choose to feed your baby is a personal decision that only you can make. Breastfeeding offers many benefits for both mother and baby that formula milk is unable to duplicate. But for those who decide that they do not want to breastfeed, formula milk provides all the nutrients a baby needs.

BENEFITS OF BREAST MILK

■ Breast milk contains the correct proportions of nutrients needed for growth and development in the first few months of life. It's the right temperature, does not need sterilizing equipment, and is free and readily available.

■ Antibodies help to protect your baby against infections such as diarrhea and vomiting, coughs and colds, and urinary and ear infections.

■ Breast milk may reduce the risk of crib death, help to prevent juvenile diabetes and protect against allergies. Some studies have found that breastfed children have better dental health, fewer bowel problems, and fewer speech problems than formula-fed babies.

■ Breastfeeding helps you develop a close bond with your baby, regain your figure more quickly, and may reduce the risk of developing breast and ovarian cancer in later life.

BREASTFEEDING TIPS

■ At the beginning of a feeding, your baby takes in low calorie "fore milk." As she continues feeding, this changes to high calorie "hindmilk." It is therefore important that your baby empties one breast before you offer her the other.

■ Let your baby feed on demand. Don't try to "build up" your supply by cutting out breastfeeding and offering formula instead. The more you feed, the more milk your breasts make.

■ The sucking action of a breastfed baby is different from that of a baby taking a bottle. When bottle feeding, the cheeks are sucked inward; with breastfeeding, the jaw muscles work rhythmically, as far back as the ears. If your baby's cheeks cave in, she is not properly attached. Don't be discouraged if your baby takes a little time to learn to latch on properly. Remember, breastfeeding is a skill to be learned and practiced.

■ If you are having difficulty, get help. The La Leche League has counselors who can help you overcome your problems (see p. 111.)

HEALTH AND DIET WHEN BREASTFEEDING

You will need about 500 extra calories a day when breastfeeding. Try to eat the balanced diet you followed during pregnancy and to include something from the four food groups daily. Three small meals are better than one large one, and have healthy snacks between meals. Don't force yourself to drink large quantities of fluid. Be guided by your body and drink when you feel thirsty.

5

BREASTFEEDING POSITIONS

Correct positioning at the breast is essential for successful breastfeeding. Otherwise, the baby will chew on your nipple, making you sore and frustrating her; it also means you will produce less milk. If she is properly positioned, she will have all of the nipple and most of the areola (the dark skin around your nipple) in her mouth.

1 Sit in a comfortable position, well supported with your baby supported in your arms, her head and shoulders facing your breast, and her nose on the same level as your nipple. Place the baby on a pillow to raise her up to the correct level if you have had a cesarean section to avoid putting stress on your scar.

2 If you are breastfeeding at night or if you find it difficult to sit because of painful stitches, you may feel more comfortable lying down. Lie down on your side with enough pillows to keep you propped up and place the baby on her side with her mouth in line with your breast.

SUCCESSFUL BOTTLEFEEDING

If you choose not to breastfeed, there is a wide choice of formula milk to choose from. To avoid infection, all equipment must be thoroughly cleaned and sterilized.

1 Wash bottles in hot soapy water, cleaning the inside with a baby brush. Rinse. Turn the nipple inside out and clean the milky film. Rinse.

2 Sterilize the bottles, disks, rings, caps, and nipples by putting them into a sterilizing solution or a steam sterilizer for the recommended amount of time, or by stacking them in the dishwasher on the hottest temperature cycle.

3 Wash your hands and make sure you have everything ready. Make the formula by boiling some fresh water and letting it cool. Measure the required amount of powder and add the formula to the correct amount of water.

4 Stir well and pour into individual bottles. Place the nipples upside down in the bottles, add the sealing caps, and shake well. Store in the refrigerator for up to 24 hours. To warm the milk, stand the bottle in a jug of hot water or an electric bottle warmer. **It is considered dangerous to heat a bottle of milk in a microwave because it will heat unevenly.** Check the temperature of the milk by dropping a little on the inside of your wrist. To feed your baby, hold her well propped up.

5

YOUR PERSONAL FILE

Although every woman experiences her pregnancy in a way that is unique for her, there are also a number of factors that are common to every pregnancy. Most pregnant women also have many questions that need answers: What symptoms should I worry about? What do I need to see me through pregnancy and to take to hospital with me? What should I buy for my baby?

The following pages are intended to help you get organized and plan ahead. This is also where important information can be kept in one place for you to find easily.

In this section you will find space to record important telephone numbers and addresses and a checklist of symptoms that make a call to your doctor a wise thing. There is also room to record appointment dates for prenatal classes and test results; and a quick reference list of what to buy for you and your baby.

6

CALLING THE DOCTOR

The majority of women go through their pregnancy without any serious health problems, but occasionally problems arise that need advice or urgent attention from a doctor. Below is a list of signs and symptoms to help you recognize early when help may be required. Some symptoms such as a mild illness may just need general advice from your doctor. Others, such as vaginal bleeding with abdominal pain, severe abdominal pain, severe itching, high blood pressure, or symptoms of preeclampsia are medical emergencies, and you should contact a doctor or hospital immediately.

SYMPTOMS REQUIRING MEDICAL ATTENTION

- Vaginal bleeding, other than light spotting.
- Signs of preeclampsia including high blood pressure; severe headache or dizziness; swelling of hands, face, or feet; blurred vision; spots before your eyes or flashing lights; vomiting in late pregnancy; large and sudden weight gain; pain in upper abdomen.
- Symptoms of an infectious disease, such as a rash or fever.
- Contact with an infectious disease to which you are not immune, such as chicken pox or rubella (German measles).
- Severe generalized itching in the last three months of pregnancy. This may be a warning sign of cholestatis of pregnancy (*obstetric cholestatis*), a rare liver disorder. Other signs may include jaundice or yellow skin, pale stools, and dark urine.
- Symptoms of a urinary tract infection including frequent passing of urine with pain, burning, or discomfort; low back pain; fever or chills; and blood in the urine.
- Abdominal pain, especially if accompanied by vaginal bleeding. In the first three months of pregnancy, severe abdominal pain accompanied by bleeding may signal a miscarriage.
- Severe vomiting.
- Signs of labor including breaking of your waters and contractions (see p. 72).
- A greenish discharge when your waters break needs urgent medical attention. Call your doctor and go to the hospital.
- Symptoms of any other infection or illness including:
    Severe sore throat
    High fever
    Swollen glands
    General fatigue or malaise with aching muscles or joint pains.
- A general feeling that "something is wrong."
- A decrease in fetal movement.

6

IN AN EMERGENCY

In the event of an emergency, there may be various people whom you or someone else will need to contact. Keep all the telephone numbers you might need in an emergency (see p.110) next to your telephone.

EMERGENCY DELIVERY IF YOU ARE ALONE

If you find that you are going into strong labor and do not have time to get to the hospital:

■ Try to stay calm. A fast labor means that your body and your baby are working well together.

■ Call for an ambulance (911) and tell them what's happening.

■ Try to find a neighbor or someone to help. Bang on a wall between apartments, open the front door and shout if you can, phone anyone who lives close by.

■ Start panting to prevent yourself from bearing down.

■ If you have time, wash your hands and vaginal area.

■ Find clean towels, a sheet, or something to wrap the baby in.

■ Try to heat the room and spread some plastic sheeting, clean sheets, towels, or newspapers on the floor, sofa or bed.

■ Lie down on these, either propped up or on your side, and wait for help.

■ If your baby arrives before help does, pant her out gently. Cradle her head while you wait for her body to emerge, but don't pull on her head. Check whether the umbilical cord is around her neck – it will feel like a thick rope. If it is, gently work it over her head. Don't tug on it.

■ Wrap your baby in whatever is available and wipe away any mucus from the nose. If necessary, clear her mouth with your finger.

■ If the cord is long enough, let your baby suck on your breast, even if you are not going to breastfeed.

■ Don't try to pull or push the placenta out. If it expels itself, wrap it up if possible and keep it at the same level as the baby.

■ Keep yourself and your baby warm under covers until help arrives.

BLEEDING IN PREGNANCY

■ Try to stay calm.

■ Call the doctor, ambulance, or hospital, or ask someone to do this for you.

■ Go to bed or lie down until help arrives.

■ Keep any bloodstained clothes; don't flush away any blood or clots until you have been seen by the doctor. Pinkish or grayish material may be pregnancy tissue and should be preserved so the doctor can check if a miscarriage is complete.

■ Don't have anything to eat or drink until the doctor tells you that it is okay.

6

PREGNANCY RECORD

These pages can be used to keep your own pregnancy diary, including important dates such as test dates and your prenatal clinic and classes appointments. You can also record how you feel physically and emotionally.

PERSONAL INFORMATION

DATE OF MY POSITIVE PREGNANCY TEST _____

DATE OF MY LAST MENSTRUAL PERIOD _____

DATE MY BABY IS EXPECTED _____

DATE I FIRST HEARD MY BABY'S HEARTBEAT _____

DATE I FIRST FELT MY BABY MOVE _____

DATE MY LABOR BEGAN _____

MY BIRTH COMPANION _____

MY BABY WAS
BORN _____   TIME _____
WEIGHT _____   LENGTH _____

MY BLOOD TYPE _____   MY PREPREGANCY WEIGHT _____

MEDICATIONS	DOSE	DATE STARTED	DATE ENDED
Folic Acid	400mg daily		

6

SPECIAL TESTS

Date	Type of procedure	Result

PRENATAL APPOINTMENTS

Date & Time	Weeks	Blood pressure	Weight	Questions to ask/comments

PRENATAL CLASSES

Name of teacher _____   Place _____

Date _____   Time _____

Special notes _____

DENTAL APPOINTMENTS

Date _____   Time _____

Date _____   Time _____

6

PREGNANCY ESSENTIALS

W hat clothes you buy during pregnancy will depend to a large extent on what you already have in your closet, what you can adapt, and your financial budget. When buying new clothes, you also need to consider the use you will get afterward, especially if you are going to breastfeed. In this case, the clothes should be front opening (see pp. 38–39 for pregnancy clothing essentials). You will also need to think about what you need to take to the hospital for you and your baby.

WHAT TO PACK FOR THE HOSPITAL

Many babies tend to arrive before they are due, so to be on the safe side have your bags packed by about 36 weeks. The hospital may give you a list of items to take in with you. If not, try to find out what the hospital provides and what you need to supply for yourself.

You may find it helpful to pack three bags – one for your hospital stay, one for labor, and a going-home bag with clothes for you and your baby. You do not need to take all the items listed. Check you have packed the essential ones, and consider what others would be useful for you, depending on your proposed length of stay.

LABOR BAG

- Sponge or facecloth for wiping your face. A natural sponge is softer than synthetic.
- Oil or lotion for your birth partner to massage you.
- Lip balm.
- Thick socks (for cold feet in labor).
- Snacks for your partner and yourself, if allowed (for example fruit, rice cakes, crackers, fruit bars, cartons of fruit juice).
- Camera and film and/or camcorder.
- A large hand mirror if you want to see your baby being born (some hospitals have mirrors, so check).
- Ties or clips for long hair.
- Waterspray or eau de cologne to cool your face.
- Cassette player and tapes.
- Nightdress or old T-shirt, if you don't want to wear a hospital gown.

FOR YOUR HOSPITAL STAY

- 1–3 nightgowns, depending on the length of your stay; these should be front opening if you are going to breastfeed.

- Light bathrobe and slippers.

- Two or three nursing/ordinary bras.

- Comfortable cotton panties.

- Washbag containing soap, facecloths, toothbrush, toothpaste, mouthwash, shampoo, deodorant, hairbrush and comb, and make-up if used.

- Washbag for birth partner with similar items.

- Wet wipes – useful for a quick wipe of your hands or face.

- Moisturizing cream/body lotion.

- Talcum powder.

- Coins and phonecard for telephone (you probably won't be able to use a cellular phone; they interfere with hospital equipment).

- Address or telephone book with essential numbers.

- Books, magazines, pen, stationery, stamps, birth announcement cards, games, knitting.

GOING-HOME BAG

Your husband could bring this in later if necessary.

- Loose comfortable clothes, such as skirt, slacks, sweater, or dress.

- Underwear, including pantyhose if necessary.

- Shoes or sandals if you have none in hospital.

- Coat or jacket if cold.

- Money for taxi if necessary.

FOR THE BABY
- Undershirt.

- 1–2 diapers.

- Stretchsuit.

- Cardigan/jacket.

- Hat.

- Blanket.

- If you are going home by car, use an approved car seat or a carrier with a fitted restraint to carry your baby. Some hospitals rent these to new parents. It is not safe to hold your baby in your arms in a moving car.

- Check what items the hospital will provide and what you need to supply yourself. Pack the necessary items in your hospital bag.

6

BABY ESSENTIALS

The list of "essentials" for your baby can seem endless, and the choice of baby goods bewildering. But although it is natural for parents to feel they want to give their baby the best of everything, you don't need to break the bank. After the baby's basic needs for love, warmth, and nourishment, material needs are few. Remember, if money is tight, your baby is not going to know whether she is bathed in a plastic bowl, the kitchen sink, or in an expensive baby bath with a stand. Or realize whether she is dressed in a designer label or hand-me-down chainstore stretchsuit. Some larger items can also be bought later or secondhand, or you may be able to borrow from friends and relatives.

GENERAL TIPS

■ Decide on your priorities: make a list of essential purchases that you will need as soon as your baby is born, a second list of what you can buy later, and a third list of luxury or optional buys.

■ If you are in doubt about buying something, wait until after the birth to see if you really need it or if you get it as a baby gift.

■ Check with friends and relatives for items to borrow, and secondhand stores and markets for bargains.

■ Collect as many store or mail-order catalogs as you can. Look through these to see what's available and compare prices. Accept trial offers of diapers and toiletries.

■ Don't buy too many first size clothes – babies soon grow out of them.

■ Think about how much space you have available at home before buying a large item such as a buggy.

BEDTIME NEEDS

■ Bassinet/portable crib or carrier. Check, if buying secondhand, that these conform to government safety standards. A bassinet should not be placed directly on the floor, so you may need a stand, too.

■ New mattress to fit the above, and conforming to government safety standards. (Recent research has found that secondhand mattresses could be a factor in some crib deaths.)

■ 4–6 flame-retardant crib sheets

■ 4–6 cotton crib blankets

■ 2 light crib covers.

BABY'S FIRST ESSENTIALS

- 4–6 cotton undershirts
- 4–6 stretch suits or 4–6 long nightgowns (low flammability)
- 2–3 cardigans/jackets
- 3–4 pairs socks or booties
- 1–2 wooly hats or summer bonnets. (If these won't stay on, wrap your baby's head in the blanket.)
- 2 pairs mittens
- 4–6 bibs
- Carrying blanket for outdoors
- Weekly supply of newborn-size disposable diapers or 24 cloth diapers and protective pants.

OTHER NEEDS

- 6 bottles, nipples, sterilizing equipment (a plastic covered container can serve as a chemical sterilizing unit), and formula milk if you are not breastfeeding.
- First car seat if you have a car.
- Toiletries such as cotton balls, mild soap, or baby wash lotion.
- Soft towel for bathing.

OPTIONAL FIRST BUYS

- Stroller
- Sling
- Baby bath
- Changing mat and changing bag
- Baby intercom.

SAFETY FIRST

- Make sure any new or secondhand equipment conforms to government safety regulations, where applicable.
- A baby does not need a pillow under the age of one.
- Make sure the mattress fits the crib/basket; don't buy secondhand.
- Quilts are not recommended for babies under the age of one, since they can overheat the baby.
- Always use a front-facing sling, rather than a back-facing one, until your baby is old enough to support her own head.

6

TELEPHONE NUMBERS

MY PARTNER CAN BE REACHED AT _____

EMERGENCY SERVICES   Tel. No: _____

FAMILY DOCTOR
Name: _____   Tel. No: _____
Address: _____

OBSTETRICIAN
Name: _____   Tel. No: _____
Address: _____

NURSE-MIDWIFE
Name: _____   Tel. No: _____
Address: _____

HOSPITAL
Name: _____   Tel. No: _____
Address: _____

NEXT OF KIN
Name: _____   Tel. No: _____
Address: _____

NEIGHBOR
Name: _____   Tel. No: _____

NEIGHBOR
Name: _____   Tel. No: _____

BABYSITTER/NURSERY/SCHOOL
Name: _____   Tel. No: _____
Address _____

HEALTH INSURANCE COMPANY
Name: _____   Tel. No: _____
Address: _____
Policy no:_____

6

USEFUL ADDRESSES

GENERAL SUPPORT OR ADVICE DURING AND/OR AFTER PREGNANCY

National Infertility Network Exchange PO Box 204 East Meadow, New York, NY 22554

American Academy of Natural Family Planning 615 S New Ballas Road, St Louis, MO 63141

Nutrition for Optimal Health Association PO Box 380, Winnetka, IL 60093

National Association of Childbearing Centers 3123 Gottschall Road, Perkiomenville, PA 18074

Healthy Mother, Healthy Babies Coalition 409 12th Street SW, Washington DC

National Eating Disorders Organization 445 E Granville Road, Worthington OH 43085

American Academy of Pediatrics PO Box 927, Elk Grove Village, IL 60009–0927

American Society for Prophylaxis in Obstetrics (ASPO)/Lamaze 1411 K Street NW Suite 200, Washington DC 20005

American Academy of Husband-Coached Childbirth PO Box 5224, Sherman Oaks, CA 91413

Post Partum Support International 927 North Kellogg Avenue, Santa Barbara, CA 93111

BREASTFEEDING

La Leche League International 140 North Meacham Road, Schaumberg, IL 60173–4840

MOTHERS OR BABIES WITH SPECIAL NEEDS

American Diabetes Association 1660 Duke Street, Alexandria, VA 22314

Epilepsy Foundation of America 4351 Garden City Drive, Landover, MD 20785

Global Maternal/Child Health Association PO Box 366, West Linn, OR 97068

March of Dimes Birth Defects Foundation 1275 Mamaroneck Avenue, White Plains, NY 10705

Leukemia Society of America 600 Third Avenue, New York, NY 10016

National Association for Down's Syndrome PO Box 4542, Oak Brook, IL 605022

Sickle Cell Disease Association of America 200 Corporate Pointe Suite 495, Culver City, CA 90230–7633

WHEN A BABY DIES

American Counseling Association 5999 Stevenson Ave, Alexandria, VA 22304–3000

SIDS Alliance 10500 Little Patuxent Parkway Suite 420, Columbia, MD 21044

Pregnancy and Infant Loss Center 1415 E Wayzata Boulevard, Wayzata, MN 53391

6

ACKNOWLEDGMENTS

t = top, *b* = bottom, *l* = left, *r* = right, *c* = center

Picture credits
5 The Stock Market; 6*t* Andrew Sydenham; 6*b* Andrew Sydenham,
Laura Wickenden; 6*br* Andrew Sydenham; 12 Laura Wickenden;
14 Jacqui Farroi/Bubbles; 15 Laura Wickenden; 16 Jo Foord; 17 Holy
Name Hospital, New Jersey; 19 Angela Hampton/Bubbles;21 Laura
Wickenden; 24*t* Laura Wickenden; 24*b* Jo Foord; 26*t* Andrew
Sydenham; 26*b* Jennie Woodcock/Bubbles; 29 Christine Hanscomb, Jo
Foord, Andrew Sydenham, Laura Wickenden; 31 Laura Wickenden;
32 Andrew Sydenham; 33 Andrew Sydenham; 34–35*t* Andrew
Sydenham; 35*b* Loisjoy Thurston/Bubbles; 38 Laura Wickenden;
39*t* Andrew Sydenham; 39*b* Laura Wickenden; 40 Laura Wickenden;
41 Andrew Sydenham; 43 Matthew Ward; 44 Jeff Hunter/The Image
Bank; 45 Matthew Ward; 48–49 Laura Wickenden; 50–51 Laura
Wickenden; 52*t* Andrew Sydenham; 52*b* Laura Wickenden; 53 Laura
Wickenden; 54*l* Iain Bagwell; 54*r* Laura Wickenden; 55 Laura
Wickenden; 56–57 Andrew Sydenham; 58 Emap Elan; 59 Laura
Wickenden; 61 Laura Wickenden; 63 Jo Foord; 65 The Stock Market;
68 The Stock Market; 68 inset The Stock Market; 73 Laura
Wickenden; 75 Laura Wickenden; 78 Laura Wickenden; 79*t* Jo Foord;
79*c* Jo Foord; 79*b* Laura Wickenden; 82 Michelle Edelmann/Bubbles;
85 Andrew Sydenham; 87 Andrew Sydenham; 89 Andrew Sydenham;
90 Laura Wickenden; 91 Frans Rombout/Bubbles; 92 Andrew
Sydenham; 93 Loisjoy Thurston/Bubbles; 94 Andrew Sydenham,
Laura Wickenden; 95 Andrew Sydenham; 96 Andrew Sydenham;
99 Andrew Sydenham; 101 Andrew Sydenham; 104 Andrew
Sydenham; 106 Laura Wickenden; 107 Andrew Sydenham; 108 The
Stock Market; 109*t* Laura Wickenden; 109*b* Andrew Sydenham

Illustration credits
13 Kevin Jones; 72 and 80 Michael Courtney; 77 and 81 Mick
Saunders; 66 and 67 Chris Forsey

REMINDERS

The first few days and weeks with a newborn are exhausting, but infinitely rewarding. This checklist will remind you of the most important points to think about.

CARING FOR YOURSELF

- Expect the first few weeks to be hectic and haphazard, and decide what your priorities are.
- Ask for pain relief if you need it.
- Get plenty of rest. Try to have a short rest while your baby is sleeping.
- Only do essential housework and limit your visitors.
- Don't feel guilty about taking time for yourself.
- Don't be a martyr. Accept any help that is offered, or if necessary, ask for it.
- If you feel you may be suffering from postpartum depression, ask for help.
- Do your pelvic floor exercises every day. Strong pelvic floor muscles help control your bladder after childbirth and are important in lovemaking.
- Watch your posture. Stand tall, stomach in, knees slightly bent.
- Always lift your baby or any other object with your knees bent.
- Change or attend to your baby on a surface that is the right height for you.
- Don't start dieting. Foods such as cereals, sandwiches, cheese, yogurt, and fruit are easy to prepare if you don't have time for cooked meals. Don't feel guilty about having take-out meals, but make sure they are as healthy as possible.
- Babies don't know what a routine is, and you will wear yourself out unnecessarily if you try to impose one.
- No parent is perfect: those who try to be feel guilty when they fail.

CARING FOR YOUR BABY

- Very few babies look perfect at birth, and most irregularities will disappear within a few weeks.
- Many mothers and fathers do not fall in love or "bond" with their baby at first; a parent-child relationship grows and matures.
- When picking up your baby or when changing, bathing, or feeding her, always hold her firmly, support her head and talk to her softly and gently, making eye contact.
- Give young brothers or sisters extra cuddles and reassurance that you still love them. Involve them in helping with the baby as much as possible.
- Correct positioning at the breast is essential for successful breastfeeding. Ask for help (over the phone if necessary) if you need it.
- The more you feed your baby, the more milk you will produce.
- If you are bottlefeeding your baby, sterilize all your equipment.

5